Crohn's Disease: Surely It Can't Happen to Me? ... I'm a Doctor

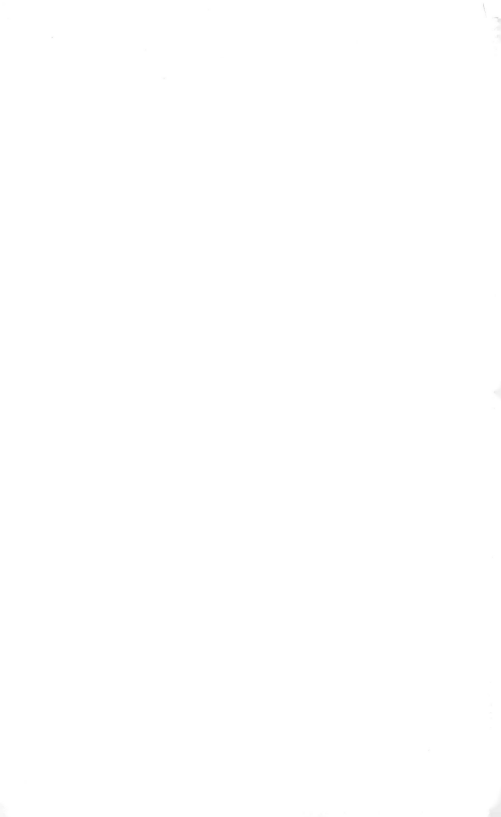

Crohn's Disease: Surely It Can't Happen to Me? ... I'm a Doctor

---

The Road to Recovery Lies Within the Diagnosis

Dr Ihsan Rashid MBChB MRCGP

ISBN: 1537730290
ISBN 13: 9781537730295

www.crohnsroadtorecovery.com
info@crohnsroadtorecovery.com

Disclaimer

ALL THE FACTUAL information that is given in my book is general information on the subject of inflammatory bowel disease (IBD) and Crohn's disease. This information is *not* a substitute for specific advice or guidance provided by your own doctor or any other healthcare professional. The products, medications, and treatments mentioned in this book are not endorsed or recommended by me. I do not accept responsibility or legal liability for any errors in the text or for the misuse or misapplication of information or material contained in this book.

Moreover, my book contains a detailed account of my own personal experience. Any adverse reactions or side effects after receiving treatment or medications are based on my own personal experience. This is intended for informational purposes only, to explain what happened to me personally, and should *not* be used to replace or undermine specific advice by your own doctor or any other professional involved in your care. Patient tolerance to medication is variable. Some individuals may tolerate medication or treatment without any significant side effects or adverse reactions, whilst others may not tolerate the same medication or treatment.

As you will read later, Crohn's disease is a very individual disease, and management is carefully tailored specifically for each individual case, instigated by your own doctor, healthcare professional, specialist, or clinician.

Acknowledgements

I WOULD LIKE to take this opportunity to thank my parents, wife, family, friends, employer, and work colleagues, who have provided so much help and support to me whilst battling through my illness with Crohn's disease.

I would also like to extend my sincere thanks to each and every healthcare professional involved in my care. I am extremely grateful for the overall high quality of health care that has been provided to me.

Contents

My Background

My name is Dr Ihsan Rashid. I am a thirty-four-year-old fully qualified medical doctor in general practice (GP) with a specialist interest in occupational health medicine. I am happily married, and my wife and I have been blessed with three beautiful children (six months, four years, and six years of age).

I was born and brought up in Scotland, United Kingdom. I have always had a passion to study medicine and become a doctor. I studied hard at secondary school to achieve the necessary grades to secure a place in medical school at university in the United Kingdom. I eventually graduated from university, gaining my medical degree (MBChB) in 2004, becoming a doctor at the age of twenty-two. Subsequently, I completed one year in hospital as a preregistration house officer (otherwise known as junior doctor), comprising a six-month surgical post followed by a six-month medical post. I then went on to complete hospital posts as a senior house officer in various specialties including accident and emergency, medicine for the elderly (coupled with acute medical receiving), psychiatry, and obstetrics and gynaecology. I wanted to pursue a career in general practice and specialised in this field, becoming a member of the Royal College of General Practitioners in early 2009.

My view is that practising as a doctor is not a right, but rather a privilege. I am privileged to be in a position where I am a health-care professional, trying to make a positive difference in my patients' health and lives.

Unfortunately, due to severe ill health pertaining to Crohn's disease, I have become a patient myself, relying on the very care that I have provided to others for years. I have struggled to sustain regular work since becoming a general-practice doctor.

I married soon after specialising in general practice. I had so much to look forward to. I had achieved so much in my career at a young age.

Unfortunately, soon after I got married, I ran into serious problems with Crohn's disease.

Nevertheless, I have remained determined to not let my disease get the better of me from either a social perspective or a career perspective. In fact, I have developed a specialist interest in occupational health medicine and commenced a training post in the private sector, in addition to my existing work in the general-practice setting.

Therefore, I have been keen to gain an extra diploma qualification in occupational health medicine and am making inroads towards this, despite my severe ill health.

Introduction

DO YOU SUFFER from inflammatory bowel disease (Crohn's disease or ulcerative colitis)?

Do you suffer from any long-standing medical conditions?

Are you looking for a method to improve your quality of life despite your illness?

Are you a medical or healthcare professional?

Do you come from a non-medical background?

Are you looking to read something unique, intriguing, and inspiring?

Do you want to read about a case that has been so complex that even medical specialists have been baffled?

If your answer to any of the above is yes, then this book will appeal to you.

I have written this book in plain, simple English, with clear explanations of medical terminology so that any person can read it, understand it, and follow me through my journey.

So many people from both medical and non-medical backgrounds have been truly inspired by my battle for survival through debilitating Crohn's disease. I have devised a strategy to help improve my recovery and quality of life.

This is not just another factual medical textbook about Crohn's disease or another typical story. This is a unique, intriguing, and inspirational real-life story about me, a fully qualified doctor, suffering from severe, complex Crohn's disease with major complications. I take you through my journey with debilitating Crohn's disease, which has led to several surgeries and put my life in danger. I explain how my skin literally became allergic to water contact—yes, that's right!

This is a book about hope and my ongoing battle for survival through extreme circumstances that could have led to breaking point. Even medical specialists have been astounded and inspired by the quality of life I have managed to achieve, given what I have had to endure.

I have relied on years of professional medical experience and, more importantly, years of personal experience as a patient to come up with a strategy that has helped my recovery and helped me to improve my quality of life profoundly.

I want to share my journey and strategy that helped me get my life back on track. I hope that other Crohn's sufferers, or indeed anybody suffering from a chronic disease, will be inspired by my story.

Through my journey, I realised that *my road to recovery actually lay within the diagnosis itself.*

You might be thinking, "How do you know what I'm going through?" I can assure you that I am in a unique position of empathising with your situation, given my experience as both a fully qualified doctor and, more importantly, a patient.

Through my battle with Crohn's disease, I have endured multiple and often prolonged and complicated hospital admissions and several surgeries, have been in a life-threatening condition, and have suffered severe and distressing symptoms subsequent to starting medical treatment. I even developed stroke-like symptoms, and my skin became allergic to water contact. I have, unfortunately, also developed degeneration (death of bone tissue) in my hips, likely secondary to medication, and at the age of thirty-four, I have been advised that I will need both my hips replaced at some point in the future. I have to live with a high-output stoma (described in chapter 1), which in itself is challenging, to say the least.

I have gathered up many years of medical experience and my experience as a patient to formulate a strategy that I adopted myself to improve my own recovery and quality of life.

This is by no means a cure or substitute for good medical care—although medical care is incorporated within my strategy. I will outline six key principles that have helped me (and I believe can help you) on the road to recovery. These principles, coupled with getting my mind around two underlying key concepts, were crucial for me to get my life back on track.

I firmly believe that adopting this strategy has helped me and will help any other patient suffering from Crohn's disease. In fact, I believe that it is applicable whether you suffer from Crohn's disease, ulcerative colitis, or any other chronic condition.

By the time you have read this book, I hope you will realise that you were staring at the solution all along in order to optimise your quality of life. I will share my discovery that the road to recovery lies within the diagnosis. All will be explained.

CHAPTER 1

Crohn's Disease: The Facts

What is Crohn's disease?

THERE IS A vast array of factual information available to us Crohn's disease sufferers. There is no doubt that if you suffer from Crohn's disease, you will be well aware of the facts.

Similarly, if you are a medical or healthcare professional, then you will also be well aware of the facts about Crohn's disease.

The purpose of my book is not to regurgitate all the factual information that is so readily available; however, I will cover some basic information on Crohn's disease in this section to enable any reader to understand the condition. In addition, throughout my story, I will explain any medical terminology as I go along so that it is easier to relate to my story.

Crohn's disease and ulcerative colitis are both forms of inflammatory bowel disease (IBD).

Crohn's disease is a condition that is essentially characterised by inflammation affecting any part of the gut. The gut is the digestive or gastrointestinal tract. Inflammation can occur anywhere in the gut, from mouth to anus (tail end/back passage). It commonly affects the last part of the small intestine/bowel (called the ileum) or large intestine (colon). It is often characterised by "skip lesions," which means that there can be segments of diseased bowel separated by segments of normal healthy bowel, almost like a sausage effect.

Crohn's disease can be very unpredictable, and its severity varies from individual to individual with some experiencing mild symptoms whilst others experience severe, debilitating, and sometimes life-threatening symptoms.

Crohn's disease follows a relapsing and remitting course. In other words, someone suffering from Crohn's disease can fluctuate between remission periods, with a few or mild symptoms, and intermittent periods of relapse (flare-ups), when symptoms become more prominent or severe. Both remission and relapse can vary in duration from days to months to even years.

Crohn's disease is a lifelong condition. Unfortunately, there is no known medical cure for this condition.

Who is affected by Crohn's disease?

Crohn's disease can affect anyone, male or female. It can occur at any age, but commonly occurs in adolescence and early adulthood. It appears to be more common among the population of people who smoke.

What are the main symptoms of Crohn's disease and why do they occur?

Rather than go into great detail about why each symptom of Crohn's disease occurs, I will outline a fundamental principle to make it easier to understand why symptoms occur.

In basic terms, our gut/gastrointestinal tract has three functions:

1. It consumes and digests the food we eat.
2. It absorbs nutrients from the food.
3. It removes waste material from our body.

This is essential for the healthy functioning not only of our bowel, but also our body as a whole. Therefore, if the gut becomes damaged or irritated, then it will not function as effectively, which can impact bowel function as well as general health.

Unfortunately, Crohn's disease causes inflammation and damage to the gut, which prevents the gut from functioning effectively. Therefore, symptoms may arise due to the direct effects of the damaged or irritated gut/digestive tract. In addition, symptoms arise due to its effect on the body as a whole.

Main symptoms include the following:

SPECIFIC SYMPTOMS

- Abdominal pain
- Diarrhoea, mixed with blood or mucus
- Mouth ulcers
- Anal fissures, small cracks or tears of the skin at the back passage (anal canal) giving rise to symptoms of severe pain and often bleeding, particularly during a bowel movement
- Haemorrhoids/piles, swelling of blood vessels in and around the anus
- Perianal abscess, a painful accumulation and collection of pus beneath the skin around the anus

3

General symptoms

- Generally feeling unwell and feverish
- Reduced appetite
- Weight loss
- Tiredness/fatigue

(Remember, Crohn's disease has a wide spectrum of potential symptoms. A Crohn's sufferer might suffer from none, some, or all of the symptoms mentioned.)

Crohn's disease can also affect other parts of the body.

Other parts of the body (outside the digestive tract) affected by Crohn's include

- blood: for example, anaemia (low blood count);
- bones/joints;
- skin;
- eyes; and
- liver.

This list is not exhaustive but gives an indication of how Crohn's disease can affect many other parts of the body, not just the gut. Once again, it is important to remember that every Crohn's disease case is individual, and cases can vary markedly in terms of type, severity, and duration of symptoms.

Are there any known causes of Crohn's disease?
The exact cause of Crohn's disease has not yet been identified; however, it is thought that it may be associated with various factors that may be interlinked.

These include the following:

- The immune system does not function properly or reacts inappropriately.
- It can run in families, indicating a possible genetic component.
- There are environmental and lifestyle factors, such as
  a. smoking;
  b. exposure to infections in the past;
  c. stress, which does not necessarily cause Crohn's disease but can be associated with a flare-up of symptoms; and
  d. certain types of diet that can be associated with worsening symptoms. (However, it has not been scientifically proven that Crohn's disease is directly caused by a particular diet.)

DISCUSSION ON CAUSES
Environmental and lifestyle factors are important for existing Crohn's disease sufferers and should be managed appropriately, as guided by your treating healthcare professional or doctor. For example, it is thought that Crohn's disease sufferers who smoke are prone to more severe symptoms, resulting in an increased risk of complications. This, in turn, increases the chances of requiring surgical intervention. Therefore, people should be encouraged to stop smoking. Similarly,

certain foods may be harmful in some individuals and trigger a relapse; therefore, this requires due care and attention.

Looking at my own situation, I suffer from Crohn's disease in one of its most aggressive forms. However, the following points are interesting:

- I am a non-smoker.
- I am the only person with Crohn's disease in my family; it does not run in the family or extended family.
- My diet has never been significantly different from that of other people who don't suffer from Crohn's disease.
- As far as I am aware, I have never been in an environment where I have been exposed to different viruses or bacteria. I am aware that, through my profession as a medical doctor, I treat people who are ill. However, there are many other doctors who have the same duties as me and do not suffer from Crohn's disease.

I think this only highlights the fact that establishing an exact cause of Crohn's disease is not that straightforward.

How is Crohn's disease investigated and diagnosed?

The diagnosis of Crohn's disease will ultimately be made by a qualified medical professional, often a gastroenterologist (a physician who specialises in diseases affecting the gastrointestinal tract, or digestive system). Whilst it is imperative to recognise symptoms and report them to your doctor as quickly as possible, it is important to refrain from self-diagnosing. Careful consideration needs to be given to the history, clinical examination, and investigative findings in order to reach a diagnosis of Crohn's disease, and this can only be done by a suitably trained and qualified doctor or specialist.

Moreover, there are other conditions that can mimic Crohn's disease or have similar symptoms or investigative findings, further highlighting the importance of diagnosis by a medical professional.

Investigations in Crohn's disease are used for diagnostic and monitoring purposes. These may include the following:

- Blood tests: These can be performed to look for evidence of anaemia (reduced red blood cell count) or raised inflammatory markers indicative of underlying inflammation or infection. Other blood tests include liver and kidney function.
- Stool tests: These are carried out to identify blood in stool, raising suspicion of Crohn's disease; to determine faecal calprotectin levels (This substance is released in excess into the intestines when inflammation is present. Therefore, this can be indicative of Crohn's disease.); or to rule out infections.
- Upper and lower gastrointestinal tract endoscopies
- Capsule endoscopy, to help with exploration of the small bowel
- Imaging, including specialised MRI and CT scans

How is Crohn's disease treated?

As mentioned earlier, there is no medical cure for Crohn's disease. Therefore, the main objective of treatment is to get symptoms under control and keep them controlled, in an attempt to improve quality of life and prevent complications. This type of management is also referred to as "inducing remission" and "maintenance treatment." This can be done using various types of medication; however, in more severe cases or cases that do not respond to medical treatment, surgical intervention may be required.

For general information purposes, I will go through some of the treatment options, which I hope will increase your understanding.

Medical Treatment
Anti-inflammatory drugs. In basic terms, these drugs are aimed at trying to reduce or dampen down the body's inflammatory response, which is thought to be the underlying mechanism giving rise to symptoms of Crohn's disease. These drugs include steroids, immunosuppressants (drugs that suppress the body's immune system, such as azathioprine and methotrexate), and biological disease-modifying agents or anti-tumour necrosis factor drugs, such as infliximab (Remicade) and adalimumab (Humira).

There is the potential for very serious complications or side effects with these potent drugs. Therefore, it is imperative that treatment is carefully managed by a specialist. Regular monitoring of blood tests and any new symptoms can be vital in ensuring safe and effective use of these drugs.

Other Treatment Options
There may also be a role for other drugs, including antibiotics, to help control Crohn's disease. Dietary treatment may also be an option; however, these options would need to be guided by your treating specialist or clinician.

Surgical Treatment
If Crohn's disease is not effectively controlled with medical treatment alone, then surgery may be required to remove segments of the intestine that have been badly damaged by inflammation. Surgery may

also be required to manage complications such as perforation of the bowel or strictures (narrowed segments of bowel).

There are various pros and cons when it comes to surgery, and these need to be considered very carefully before opting for surgical treatment.

Whilst surgery can be potentially life-saving and can help alleviate some of the symptoms of Crohn's disease, it is still *not* curative. In other words, Crohn's disease can keep recurring again and again, causing significant damage to previously healthy tissue of the gut. This was apparent in my own case, as you will read about later. Therefore, Crohn's disease still requires careful management, often with medication, even after surgery in an attempt to keep it under control.

USING A STOMA

Treatment for Crohn's disease can sometimes require formation of a stoma. This is basically a surgical procedure in which an opening is created in the front of the abdomen allowing the end of the intestine to be brought out. This, in turn, creates a diversion allowing waste products from the digestive process to be redirected into a pouch (bag) as opposed to eliminating via the anus (back passage).

A stoma that is formed using the lowest part of the small intestine is called an ileostomy.

A stoma that is formed using the large intestine is called a colostomy.

The waste material that accumulates in an ileostomy bag needs to be drained or disposed of up to six times daily; however, this can vary depending on the type of bag used. The ileostomy appliance or flange (which is stuck on to the skin of the abdomen) will also need to be removed and replaced at regular intervals, which can also vary, again, depending on the type of appliance used.

Having a stoma can have a significant impact on your life. In my experience, it can take months or even up to a year to learn how to effectively manage a stoma and incorporate it into your life. I will explain later in chapters 2 and 3 how having a stoma (ileostomy) affected me and the challenges I faced.

What complications can arise from Crohn's disease?
Complications of Crohn's disease may include the following:

- Strictures, narrowed segments of bowel that can obstruct the flow of food through the intestine, resulting in severe abdominal pain and vomiting
- Fistula, an abnormal connection between the diseased bowel and other bowel loops or internal organs (Abnormal connections can also occur between the diseased bowel and external skin around the back passage [anus].)
- Perforations, where the bowel ruptures or perforates, resulting in an opening or hole (This creates a pathway for faecal waste material to leak out into the abdomen, resulting in severe infection or abscess formation. This can be life-threatening.)
- Adverse effects to medication, such as steroids
- Malnourishment
- Slightly higher risk of developing bowel cancer

What is the long-term outlook for the patient?

Crohn's disease is a very unpredictable life-long condition that follows a relapsing and remitting course, as previously explained. Periods of relapse and remission can vary significantly from days to months to even years. There is no set pattern and every case is individual. There is wide variation in patient experience with this condition, and response to and tolerance of treatment are also varied.

On one end of the spectrum, some people with mild symptoms may not require much in the way of medical intervention and are able get on with their daily tasks of living with minimal disruption. However, on the other end of the spectrum, some people may experience severe, relentless symptoms despite treatment, causing major disruptions to their day-to-day living.

I will talk later about how I improved my quality of life whilst living with severe debilitating Crohn's disease.

CHAPTER 2

How I Have Been Affected by Crohn's Disease: My Complex Story

IT HAS BEEN difficult even for my treating clinicians to fully comprehend what has happened to me. Although I now have a clear diagnosis of Crohn's disease, initially it was tricky to come to a definitive diagnosis.

I was a young, fit, and active medical doctor with no previous significant health issues. Before I knew it, I became one of the most complex medical cases that some of my treating medical healthcare professionals had come across. The hospital has, unfortunately, become like a second home to me, with countless admissions, extensive investigations, including MRI and CT scans, and repeated surgery, including emergency life-saving surgery.

Although I suffer from a severe form of Crohn's disease, my story does not stop there. I have had to endure severe, sometimes unexplained, adverse reactions after commencing treatment. Some investigative findings have even put a question mark over my diagnosis at times. This, along with various other complicating factors, has made it very difficult to establish maintenance treatment to control the disease in my case.

Please do not worry if it sounds like a lot to take in as you read on—you are not the only one! I will explain every piece of medical terminology as I go along to help you understand my case. After reading my story, you will undoubtedly gain insight into the severe difficulties that I have encountered.

Also, please remember that my book is not just about my story but is also about a unique strategy that I have developed to help improve my own quality of life and get my life back on track, having relied on years of professional medical experience and experience as a patient. It may sound like a cliché, but I feel that this will prove that there is always light at the end of the tunnel. I hope that this will be an inspiration to all Crohn's disease sufferers, and indeed anyone suffering from any form of inflammatory bowel disease or other chronic medical illness.

So here goes—this is my story:

I started to experience symptoms of diarrhoea, rectal bleeding (bleeding from the back passage), abdominal pain, and severe anorectal spasm (spasm of muscles at the back passage) soon after completing my specialty training in general practice. I frequently noticed blood in the toilet after a bowel movement. I was spending longer and longer time in the toilet and had excruciating pain after bowel movements. The pain would last up to six to seven hours, rendering me housebound and immobile at times. My symptoms were progressively worsening. It was affecting my ability to work, and going about my tasks of daily living became increasingly difficult. I was struggling to spend quality time with my family due to the severity of my symptoms.

Being a doctor, I obviously knew that something was not right and therefore visited my own GP. I was referred to a specialist in the hospital, and after further investigations including upper gastrointestinal endoscopy, colonoscopy, and MRI of my small bowel, I was diagnosed with Crohn's disease.

Unfortunately, by the time my Crohn's disease was diagnosed, I had already developed several strictures in my small bowel. A stricture is a narrowed segment of intestine that can result in obstruction of the flow of food, resulting in severe abdominal pain and vomiting.

Even having one stricture is a significant complication of Crohn's disease, but I had developed five strictures at the time of diagnosis.

I was started on a course of steroids to help dampen down the inflammation in my bowel in the acute (short-term) phase, and I was given various topical creams to apply to the tail end to help with pain from what was thought to be anal fissures (tears in the lining of the anal canal, resulting in pain and bleeding, worse during a bowel movement).

Unfortunately, I developed some horrible side effects to the steroids. My face began to swell up, and I developed pain and swelling in the temporal regions of my head (the side of the head behind the eyes) when eating. This meant that after a few bites of food, my face would feel too painful to continue eating. Whilst a puffy face is a known side effect of steroids, the painful swelling in my temples when eating was unusual. I felt embarrassed to eat in front of other people. I would struggle to open and close my jaw after a few bites of food, and my temple regions would swell up like small balloons, causing significant discomfort. My Crohn's symptoms were already affecting my social life, and this horrible side effect made matters worse. I ended up requiring repeated courses of oral steroids throughout the course of my illness, which also caused difficulty in sleeping. This had the effect of making me even more tired the following day. I suffered from anaemia (low blood count) which made me feel fatigued and exhausted at the best of times.

Despite steroid medication, I was really struggling with symptoms of severe prolonged spasm affecting the back passage after a bowel movement. It sounds embarrassing, but it was traumatic. My family, unfortunately, were used to seeing me lie down for hours on end in severe pain, waiting for the symptoms to subside. Even changing posture, for example trying to stand up from a sitting position, would make the spasm pain ten times worse. Painkillers and topical creams would not ease the pain. I basically had to lie still for hours and let it calm down itself. This happened every time following a bowel movement. It was very distressing, to say the least, and you can only imagine the difficulties this caused in my day-to-day living.

Eventually, I was referred to the surgical team for further investigation of this spasm pain. I underwent an examination under anaesthetic as a day case. This was meant to be for investigation and diagnostic purposes only. However, due to the severity of spasm evident on examination, I received an injection of Botox in the tail end to try to alleviate my symptoms.

On waking from this procedure, I woke up shivering and hypothermic (low body temperature). I had to be wrapped in special equipment to help raise my body temperature. I also became wheezy and several times required nebulisation (inhaling medication as a mist into the lungs through a face mask, a common form of emergency medication used to provide relief from symptoms of severe asthma, which typically manifests with shortness of breath and wheeze). I also required potent medication to control the pain from the back passage.

After returning home from the hospital on this particular occasion, I experienced side effects of nausea, vomiting, and headaches due to the medication. The side effects resolved or settled down eventually.

Furthermore, I had extremely low iron levels (which can be common in Crohn's disease), resulting in feeling very fatigued and tired. I could not tolerate oral iron supplements due to the side effects. Therefore, arrangements were made for me to be admitted to the hospital to receive an iron infusion. I could not have imagined what was about to happen.

I made myself comfortable in my hospital bed. I was expecting to be admitted for a short period of time to receive my iron infusion. I did not really think much of it, and I was already planning what I was going to do after the infusion. Intravenous access was gained so that the iron infusion could be delivered directly into my bloodstream. Within ten to fifteen seconds of starting the infusion, whilst the nurse was present, I felt very nauseated and started retching. I asked for a sick bowl. I developed sudden excruciating chest pain radiating to my back. I had tears flowing down my face, and I was screaming in agony with chest pain. The infusion was stopped immediately and doctors rushed to the scene. There were concerns that I had suffered an allergic reaction, but in fact, it turned out that I had developed coronary vasospasm.

Coronary vasospasm is a sudden, intense tightening in one or more of the major arteries supplying blood to the heart muscle. It can cause severe chest pain, abnormalities in heart rhythm, and even death.

Eventually, the pain settled. I was kept overnight for observation. I was not allowed to have an iron infusion again. I have had ongoing problems with iron deficiency throughout my illness with Crohn's disease. Unfortunately, I cannot tolerate iron supplements, therefore treatment is limited for me.

In the early stages of my diagnosis, I remember many occasions of having to phone in sick at work. There were times when I woke up in the morning, felt all right, and got myself ready for work. However, just when I was ready to leave the door I had to run to the toilet, and then I was in too much pain to go to work. There were times when symptoms started while I was at work, and I had to leave early as I was too unwell to continue. There were even times when I was en route to work but had to turn back due to my symptoms. In my line of work, phoning in sick causes major disruptions, as it can be difficult to get another doctor to cover at such short notice. As I am sure you are already aware, surgeries and clinics are very busy and often fully booked. Therefore, a cancellation can result in many patients, as well as staff, becoming frustrated at having to reschedule if there is no doctor available. I would always feel guilty if I had to call in sick, but it was really out of my control. Crohn's disease is so unpredictable, and symptoms can flare at any time without warning.

I was newly married when I started to develop symptoms of Crohn's disease. I felt as if my life was starting to revolve around the toilet. I remember a constant struggle with my bowel habit and pain. However, my wife has always stood by me and has been incredibly supportive through some extreme circumstances, which you will read about later in my story. I remain so grateful to her. We are happily married, with three beautiful children, and I would not change it for anything in this world.

Hospital Admissions in 2012

Despite my ill health, I still wanted to excel in my career and establish some stability in my life, especially with an expanding family. I had an interview in 2012 for an exciting job as a salaried general practitioner. Despite some tough competition, I was contacted with a job offer within hours of my interview. The GP practice was keen to take me on board. I was delighted to accept. The job was located in England, which meant that I would have to relocate with my family. At the point when I accepted the job offer, my Crohn's symptoms appeared to have calmed down somewhat, as I was tapering off the steroids. I remained optimistic that things were settling, therefore I was happy to accept the job offer and remained very excited by this new job opportunity allowing me to further progress in my career as a doctor.

I remained committed to making this work. I made several trips down to England to find a place to live at short notice. Moving to a new city was challenging. However, after a lot of time, effort, driving to and from, packing and unpacking, lifting and shifting, we eventually moved into our new home in England. I wanted to make sure my wife was comfortable, as she was pregnant with our second child at the time. I breathed a sigh of relief once we had shifted and moved into our new home. I remember thinking I will not be moving house again for a long time. It was hard work!

Unfortunately, just after commencing my new job in England, my Crohn's symptoms flared up. It turned out that I was only able to sustain work in my new job for those initial few weeks. This was just the start of falling so seriously unwell that I would be out of work for several months. You can imagine how deeply unsettling this was for me, my pregnant wife, and our two-year-old daughter at the time. I was devastated that I had to let the new position go. I would have to move my family back up to Scotland. Moving house is difficult as it is, but arranging this while remaining unwell was even more difficult. I had no option.

So here's what happened in a little more detail. Just after commencing my new job in England, I started to develop diarrhoea with bleeding and pain at the back passage despite recent treatment with steroids. I contacted my gastroenterologist, and I was started on azathioprine (an immunosuppressant medication commonly used in Crohn's disease to dampen the body's overactive immune response in an attempt to reduce inflammation) for the first time in 2012. It had been extremely difficult to establish me on any form of maintenance medication, as you will read about later.

In the days after starting azathioprine, I started to notice a mild headache. I initially thought that it was perhaps due to eye strain in relation to using the computer at work. I made an appointment with the optician and was noted to not have any major issues with my vision.

A few weeks after starting azathioprine (and only a few weeks into my new job), I woke up one morning sweating profusely, with a severe pounding headache and severe chest pain.

I visited the local accident and emergency department, where they were more concerned about the chest pain. After excluding a cardiac-related issue, I was discharged shortly after.

Unfortunately, only days after the previous admission and still within weeks of starting azathioprine, my symptoms worsened to the extent that an ambulance was called, and I was rushed to the hospital.

Subsequently, I was admitted to the hospital medical ward via accident and emergency, initially with suspected meningitis (a life-threatening condition that can kill in hours if not treated rapidly) or subarachnoid haemorrhage (bleeding in the brain). The headaches and chest pain were severe. I was not sure what was happening initially. All I knew was that I felt very ill. My family were also deeply concerned.

In the accident and emergency department, I had an emergency CT scan to exclude a bleed in the brain. This was thankfully excluded; however, a small lesion in my brain was noted. This was also noted on a previous MRI scan of my head. The exact nature of this lesion was unknown, but at that moment, it was thought to be unrelated to my severe headaches.

I was treated with strong antibiotics administered intravenously (through my veins) in case I had developed meningitis, fluid drips, and pain relief medication in the accident and emergency department. Subsequently, I was transferred to a medical ward, where I remained overnight. I received a lumbar puncture (a medical procedure that involves inserting a needle into the lower part of the spine to extract fluid) the next day to help completely exclude a bleed in the brain and also to test for signs of meningitis.

This brought back memories of when I first performed this procedure on one of my own patients when I was a junior doctor more than a decade ago. I remembered a sense of achievement when I became competent in this procedure. I thought that I had no idea at the time that the roles would be reversed in the future, when I was to become the patient undergoing this procedure. Every step in the hospital would be so familiar for me; however, the familiarity was due to having worked in this very environment as a doctor for so many years. My experience as a patient, therefore, was somewhat surreal.

Thankfully, the test came back as clear, although my blood tests continued to indicate that I had a serious infection going on somewhere.

I was obviously very concerned about my severe headaches, and it seemed highly coincidental that this had developed so soon after starting azathioprine.

During this admission in 2012, I remained symptomatic with chest pains. To make matters worse, a troponin blood test came back as strongly positive. This is a blood test that, if positive, can indicate damage to the heart muscle, as found in heart attacks. I was thinking, "what is going on?"

Following review by a consultant cardiologist, I was transferred to the coronary-care unit for close monitoring, and I required an urgent echocardiogram (ultrasound scan of the heart), which was done on the ward. Thankfully, there was no significant heart damage noted on the echocardiogram. I remained in the coronary-care unit for several days during this admission for further tests and monitoring. Whilst in coronary care, I was also reviewed by another specialist, who advised further blood tests and continued treatment for possible meningitis. Once stable, I was transferred from coronary care to the cardiology ward, in view of persistent chest-pain symptoms. I was eventually diagnosed with myocarditis, which is an inflammation of the heart muscle. This explained the persistent chest pain that I was experiencing.

Unfortunately, the severity of my headaches worsened, and I was reviewed by a neurologist on the cardiology ward. It became evident that I had developed a weakness affecting the entire left side of the body, which may have been suggestive of a stroke. It was noted that I had persistent severe headaches requiring very potent medication to try to control the pain. The neurologist was concerned and arranged for immediate transfer to the neurology ward, where I stayed for the remainder of this admission. I remember being transferred in the middle of the night to the other side of the hospital. I felt scared and apprehensive. I was only too well aware of the implications of a stroke, if this was diagnosed. I felt helpless. I felt as if I was not in control of what was happening to my body. This did not seem like reality. Surely this could not be happening to me?

I went on to receive several MRI scans (head, neck, and thoracic spine) to rule out any problems in my neurological system. Thankfully, the results came back as normal.

As you can imagine, this hospital admission in 2012 was a very concerning time for me. I had initially suspected meningitis, which is potentially a life-threatening condition if not treated quickly and adequately. There were then concerns of a cardiac (heart) event, resulting from raised troponin, commonly seen in patients with a heart attack. To make matters worse, I then developed neurological symptoms that could have been suggestive of a stroke. My treating clinicians and I were wondering what was going on. I had symptoms suggestive of three potentially life-threatening conditions during the same admission in 2012.

I remained on a cocktail of medications, including morphine-based medication.

There was no clear explanation for my symptoms. I had developed a multisystem inflammatory response affecting my cardiovascular and neurological systems. In addition, I had a small lesion in my brain. Again, there was no clear diagnosis, despite countless blood tests and specialised scans, including CT and MRI scans. However, blood tests did reveal very high inflammation levels, indicating that there was a serious infection going on somewhere. I was seriously ill, but even my treating clinicians were somewhat confused by my symptoms.

I actually did not have any significant Crohn's disease symptoms during this hospital admission. Perhaps the symptoms were masked by the potent medications I was on. Prior to discharge, I underwent a colonoscopy (a test using a thin, flexible tube to visualise the large intestine) to check on my Crohn's disease. The biopsies (analysis of small samples of body tissue) were consistent with chronic inflammatory bowel disease.

I was discharged with ongoing unexplained symptoms (severe headaches and chest pains) that had started after commencing treatment with azathioprine. Due to the complexity and severity of my case, I required outpatient follow-up with various specialties, including cardiology, gastroenterology, and neurology.

Following discharge, my recovery was very prolonged and challenging. I had ongoing problems with chest pain and shortness of breath on exertion. After consultation with my cardiologist, I underwent further tests, in the form of an exercise tolerance test and CT angiogram, to ensure that there was no evidence of coronary heart disease. Thankfully, these were normal, and it was thought that I was suffering from prolonged myocarditis (inflammation of the heart muscle).

After being discharged from the hospital on this occasion, I also continued to suffer persistent, severe headaches affecting the back of my head. I remained on morphine-based medication for this, but I was pretty much bedbound with these symptoms. I spent up to eight hours per day lying down with severe headaches, despite strong medication. These symptoms persisted for approximately six months. For six months, I was crippled with severe headaches and continued to suffer cardiac symptoms of chest pain and shortness of breath on exertion.

I could not function with these severe headaches. The symptoms were relentless. I was out of work for so long that I had financial concerns and concerns about how I would be able to sustain work in the future. I had my new job at the back of my mind, wondering whether I would be able to return to it. It turned out that I would not be fit to return to my new job, or any job, for a further six months. Those were very difficult times.

I was inundated with hospital appointments and investigations, scan after scan. Subsequent tests, including an MRI scan, which continued to show a lesion in my brain, also raised the question of tuberculosis (TB), which is a serious bacterial infection. Unlike Crohn's disease, TB can be treated and cured.

As a precautionary measure, I was started on treatment for one full year in an attempt to treat for possible TB infection, although there was never a definitive diagnosis of TB. This, in itself, was difficult. For one full year, every single day without fail, I had to take strong TB medication coupled with extremely high doses of oral steroids, which caused a recurrence of severe side effects, as previously mentioned. I could not sleep, my face was swollen, and I could not chew my food due to facial pain. I felt like my whole body system was upside down; however, I persevered and remained compliant with my medications.

There were also questions as to whether I was actually suffering from TB as opposed to Crohn's disease. Although intestinal tuberculosis is rare in Western countries, its clinical presentation can mimic Crohn's disease, making the diagnosis difficult to establish.

My underlying diagnosis was up in the air, and for some time I even put it down to gastrointestinal TB, since my bowel symptoms had taken a back seat during this period. I also recall one of the reports of a small-bowel MRI raising the question of whether I had TB rather than Crohn's. I was actually hoping that my diagnosis was gastrointestinal TB, because there is curative treatment for TB (which effectively means that I could have been cured), unlike Crohn's disease, for which there is no known medical cure, requiring lifelong treatment with potent medication. For some time, many of us were scratching our heads, thinking, what's the diagnosis?

I was concerned about recommencing maintenance treatment for Crohn's disease based on previous experience with azathioprine and risk of intracerebral (brain) infection, and also due to the uncertainty of diagnosis at this point. I did not want treatment for Crohn's disease if this was not my diagnosis.

As previously mentioned, azathioprine is an immunosuppressant that dampens the immune system, making it more difficult to fight infection. Therefore, in view of this unexplained lesion in my brain (which may have been infective in origin), there was a risk of potentially life-threatening infection if my immune system was dampened, and I was not able to fight infection well.

It may appear, so far in my story, that my bowel symptoms were somewhat overshadowed by the severe difficulties I faced after commencing different medications for a period of time. However, while many symptoms remained unexplained at the time, one thing was for sure, looking at things retrospectively: I was suffering from an underlying severe form of Crohn's disease affecting my small bowel, and it was just waiting to erupt.

The delay in starting maintenance treatment for Crohn's disease (due to the complexity of my case and no one's fault) would prove very significant indeed.

Hospital Admissions in 2013

Despite one full year of TB treatment, the strictures flared up again, resulting in several further hospital admissions with symptoms suggestive of bowel obstruction. A bowel obstruction occurs when the bowel becomes blocked (in my case as a result of strictures), resulting in severe abdominal pain and vomiting.

The recurrence of my symptoms made it apparent that I was definitely suffering from Crohn's disease as opposed to TB, since the previous TB treatment should have cured me.

As mentioned, I had repeated hospital admissions with severe abdominal pain. My family were distressed watching me in so much pain. The pain was excruciating, requiring high doses of morphine to control it. My symptoms were managed conservatively with medical treatment. Unfortunately, after several admissions with severe abdominal pain in quick succession, it was evident that I was not responding to medical treatment, including steroids. Further MRI scans revealed that the strictures had become fibrotic, or permanently scarred. This meant that no medication could reverse the strictures that were causing the severe abdominal pain.

I had no option but to undergo a major bowel surgery in late 2013. I mentally prepared myself that I would require maintenance treatment for Crohn's disease after recovering from surgery.

This was the first time in my life that I was about to undergo major surgery. I was fully aware of the protocols and procedures involved. However, this familiarity was from a doctor's perspective, not from being a patient myself. I was able to explain the surgery, as well as the risks, to my family. I was apprehensive but remained optimistic that it would all work out. I really did not have any choice.

As I lay in my hospital bed waiting to be taken to the operating room for surgery, the whole experience felt surreal. I had previous experience assisting in surgical procedures during my training many years ago and was so familiar with being on the other side, as a doctor ensuring that my patients were ready for their surgery and caring for them postoperatively. Even writing my signature on the consent form felt surreal. I usually would be signing on the dotted line next to "Doctor's Signature," but on this occasion the roles were reversed, and I signed next to "Patient's Signature." This was an invaluable experience for me, to fully understand the importance of helping put patients at ease prior to undergoing any type of procedure. Here I was a fully qualified doctor, yet I remained anxious about what was going to happen.

I eventually underwent the major bowel surgery to correct the five strictures (blockages) in my small bowel and to remove a segment of diseased bowel.

Unfortunately, postoperatively, I developed a pelvic abscess. This is basically a collection of infected fluid inside the pelvis. It is a serious condition that can occur following abdominal surgery and requires careful monitoring and treatment.

I could feel painful pressure within my pelvis. This caused me to cry out loud in pain and prolonged my hospital admission even further. The pelvic abscess was another barrier to commencing maintenance treatment. In fact, I remember my gastroenterologist coming to the surgical ward after my operation, looking to start me on maintenance treatment. However, the gastroenterologist was disappointed to discover that I had developed a pelvic abscess and therefore could not start treatment.

Maintenance treatment for Crohn's disease generally involves use of drugs that weaken or dampen the body's natural immune system, therefore making it more difficult to fight infection. If the immune system is weakened while there is an active pelvic infection (or any infection), then this can result in worsening infection and potentially life-threatening complications. Therefore, it was too risky and dangerous to begin maintenance treatment at this time; hence it was put on hold.

I was treated aggressively with intravenous antibiotics (three different types of antibiotics simultaneously) for the pelvic abscess.

Moreover, I had a small leakage of discharge from the bottom of my wound. Therefore, the surgeons had to undo some of the superficial stitches to allow this infection to drain.

I remained on oral antibiotics after discharge and required several CT scans to ensure that the pelvic abscess was resolving.

Eventually, following surgery, I recovered to the extent that I was able to return to some level of function. My understanding is that pathology (examination under a microscope) of the segment of bowel cut out during surgery was essentially normal. This was somewhat surprising. I expected it to clearly show evidence of Crohn's disease, especially as I could recall my surgeon mentioning that the resected segment of bowel was inflamed and swollen. This raised the question, once again, of whether or not these strictures were in fact a result of Crohn's disease.

Unfortunately, a few months later, I started to develop severe abdominal pains again after eating, along with some diarrhoea and rectal bleeding with severe spasms. The recurrence of symptoms more or less confirmed that I was definitely suffering from Crohn's disease as opposed to gastrointestinal TB, despite the question marks raised along my journey. As mentioned earlier, this was also in view of the fact that I should have been cured with the year-long TB treatment that I had received.

I went on to have various ups and downs and required oral ste-roids intermittently for acute flare-ups of Crohn's disease. I had to endure the horrible side effects of steroid medication every time I was on it. There were many nights that I struggled to sleep due to the ef-fects of the steroids.

I had a further discussion with my gastroenterologist. We agreed to try a nutritional diet to try to control my symptoms, as opposed to other immunosuppressant medication. Other forms of maintenance treatment were thought to be too risky due to the risk of intracerebral (brain) infection, especially as a further scan of my brain had revealed some change around the unknown lesion. I still had apprehensions about restarting immunosuppressant medication again, which was completely understandable in view of my past ex-perience with azathioprine. Therefore, the nutritional diet seemed a good option, given the complexity of my case and no significant risk of side effects. However, this form of treatment came with its own set of challenges.

I was referred to a dietician and commenced on an exclusive Modulen IBD treatment diet for approximately six weeks with a view to gradual reintroduction of food.

Modulen IBD treatment is a special nutritional diet. It comes in powdered form that is mixed with water to make it into a drink. It's similar to a milkshake in consistency. It can be used exclusively (without eating any food) and will meet daily nutritional require-ments. It is taken under careful supervision and guidance of a spe-cialist and dietician. It is used to help treat symptoms of Crohn's disease.

However, this was such an incredibly difficult time for me. Not being able to eat affected both my family and social life. Food has always been something I have enjoyed, and to avoid this was almost impossible, but I persevered. I actually felt as if I was starving, and no amount of Modulen satiated my hunger. This made me very upset. It made me realise that it was virtually impossible to remain on this diet long term. There was some improvement in symptoms initially, but I started to develop abdominal pain again, with associated diarrhoea and rectal bleeding. However, no clear specific food was identified as the trigger. From my perspective, nutritional treatment was neither fully successful nor viable for me.

As mentioned earlier, my case was so complicated and ambiguous that maintenance treatment was difficult to establish, through no one's fault. It is just the way things worked out.

I had no idea what was going to happen to me next. If I thought that things could not get worse, then I was sadly mistaken. Unfortunately, I was soon to realise that my Crohn's disease was going to hit me even harder and eventually lead to developing life-threatening complications come 2015.

Year 2015: The Most Difficult Time of My Life

The year 2015 was the most difficult, challenging, and traumatic time of my life. It was equally traumatic for my family.

I went on a road trip to England with my wife and two children. We were really looking forward to our trip, as we were visiting family, and it had been a while since we had been on a family trip. We drove down to England to spend a few days with family and enjoy an outing. We drove quite far south, stopping along the way to meet family. We enjoyed meeting with our family. The weather was really nice, and we had a very enjoyable time.

I was now focused on returning home in preparation for work after the holiday weekend. We left England to drive back home to Scotland. I had booked a hotel stopover to spend the night, to break the journey, and make driving more enjoyable and easier.

As we left England, night had fallen, and it was quite wet and windy. We felt relieved that we were only driving for two hours to the hotel, as opposed to driving all the way up to Scotland, which would have taken approximately five hours.

En route, I started to feel a niggling discomfort in my abdomen, which I thought was a bit of indigestion, as we had a late meal before departing. I managed to bear the discomfort, and we arrived at our hotel. I felt the need to relieve my bladder on arrival, which I thought would help ease the discomfort. I was wrong.

I came out of the bathroom and told my wife that I did not feel well. Thankfully, the children were tired from the journey and fast asleep in bed. Within minutes, my abdominal discomfort turned into pain, and then the pain became agony. Before I knew it, I was crying out in agony. The pain was coming in waves and became more and more intense. Tears were flowing from my eyes. I told my wife to ask reception to call an ambulance.

The hotel staff and manager rushed to the scene, at which point I was rolling in agony. An ambulance arrived shortly after; however, I was in too much distress to be transported out of the room into the ambulance. The paramedics gained intravenous access and administered a high dose of morphine directly into my bloodstream. This eventually provided enough pain relief that I could be transferred to the ambulance. I was rushed to the nearest accident and emergency department, leaving my wife and children at the hotel. I was also concerned about my family. We had no family near our location at the time.

Subsequently, I was admitted to the hospital in early April 2015. I underwent further blood tests, x-rays, and a CT scan of my abdomen. The CT scan was reported as showing signs of inflammation due to Crohn's disease.

I was yet again commenced on a reducing course of steroids (starting at high dose and gradually tapering down). My father and sister had to drive to our location in England to support my wife and children and help drive them back to Scotland. I was too unfit to be driven back to Scotland. I took a flight back immediately after being discharged from hospital.

What was intended to be an enjoyable family trip turned out to be a nightmare. I remained on oral steroids at this point, and the abdominal pain subsided. I thought that perhaps the acute flare-up was over. Again, I was wrong.

Unfortunately, this was just the beginning.

After arriving back in Scotland, I began to suffer diarrhoea, rectal bleeding, and severe spasm pain at the back passage once again. Abdominal pain was not the predominant symptom at this point. Oral steroids were not working. After discussion with my gastroenterologist, I was admitted to the hospital to receive a course of intravenous steroids.

This hospital admission with a further flare-up of Crohn's was only weeks after the last admission in England in April 2015. I remained optimistic that, on this occasion, it was going to be a short admission for treatment to control the acute flare-up, but I was wrong. Despite being treated aggressively with intravenous steroids, I also developed symptoms of severe abdominal pain again while in the hospital. This abdominal pain was severe and colicky in nature (coming in waves), getting worse after eating.

As a result of steroid treatment, I suffered from massive generalised swelling, especially of my legs. I put on approximately twelve kilograms of weight in as many days, mainly due to fluid accumulating in my body. I could barely recognise myself in the mirror. I could not even properly feel my own legs due to the swelling. The pain was so severe that I was crying out loudly in pain. Once again, I required potent medication to control my pain.

I feared the worst, that I had developed strictures in my small bowel again due to the fact that the pain felt so similar.

I was too unwell for a small-bowel MRI, as it required drinking Klean Prep for better visualization of the bowel. For those who do not know, this is a foul-tasting liquid preparation that is extremely difficult to even smell, let alone drink, and I had to drink two jugs of it before the MRI scan. It causes loose bowel movements for several hours afterward, which can potentially cause dehydration.

After receiving approximately two weeks of high-dose intravenous steroids in the hospital, I was deemed stable to undergo a specialised MRI scan to check my small bowel for strictures. In view of my persistent severe abdominal pain, I was somewhat surprised that the MRI did not show any strictures and was reported as clear. On the one hand, this was great news, as it meant that the need for surgery was much less likely, but on the other hand, it really made us wonder what was causing such severe pain, which was so similar to the pain I had experienced when I previously had strictures.

Why did the detailed MRI scan not reveal any abnormality?

Perhaps the aggressive intravenous steroid treatment had worked?

Perhaps there were inflammatory strictures that had reversed with the aggressive intravenous steroid treatment?

In simple terms, an inflammatory stricture is a narrowed segment of bowel due to active inflammation. It can be reversed by treating with anti-inflammatory medication such as steroids. A fibrotic stricture refers to a narrowed segment of bowel that has become permanently scarred, and it is not reversible with medical treatment. Therefore, fibrotic strictures usually require surgical treatment.

Sometimes strictures can be caused by a combination of both.

However, this did not explain why my severe abdominal pain persisted. If the presumed inflammatory strictures had resolved, surely my severe abdominal pain after eating should have resolved as well.

I was puzzled, as I still required high doses of intravenous morphine to control my pain, which occurred after eating and was of the exact same character and intensity as what I suffered when I had confirmed strictures in the past. For this reason, I had a surgical review. My surgeon understandably did not wish to operate, especially in view of the normal MRI scan result. I was pleased and thought perhaps it might resolve with medication. I was placed on a liquid diet with a view to gradual reintroduction to food. I was also started on an atypical type of medication for the pain.

During this admission, I started to become short of breath and fatigued. My haemoglobin level (blood count) dropped so low that I required a blood transfusion. I developed some cardiovascular symptoms such as chest pain as well. I was investigated further via twenty-four-hour heart monitor, electrocardiogram (tracing of heart rhythm) and echocardiogram (ultrasound scan of the heart). The echocardiogram reported some fluid around my heart (pericardial effusion), to add to my worries. I was subsequently referred for a cardiology review. Thankfully, I was reassured and given the all-clear by a cardiologist.

To make matters worse, I developed further bleeding from the back passage during this admission and went for a colonoscopy. There were some mild changes noted on colonoscopy, but nothing too significant.

Despite being heavily sedated during the colonoscopy, I was informed later that I was jumping off the table during the procedure due to the severity of my pain.

My gastroenterologist was now concerned that I may also be suffering from visceral hypersensitivity. This refers to the condition when the internal organs are hypersensitive to pain. It can be quite common in irritable bowel syndrome (IBS) sufferers. If you suffer from visceral hypersensitivity, then an internal issue that would not usually cause any problems manifests as pain, often severe in nature.

So I thought, maybe this explains my severe abdominal pain in the absence of any MRI scan findings.

My symptoms had not resolved, but I was discharged home (after four long weeks in the hospital) on a reducing dose of steroids and morphine-based medication to take as required for pain. I was also advised to take a higher dose of a new medication (an atypical agent) in an attempt to control the pain. Here's a long list of my medications on this particular discharge to give you some insight into the extent of treatment that I required:

- Calceos, to supplement calcium and vitamin D
- Chlorphenamine (Piriton), to control itch from steroids
- Dermol 500 lotion, to moisturise dry, cracked skin
- Diltiazem 2 percent cream, applied to back passage for healing of anal fissure
- E45 cream, a moisturiser
- Folic acid
- Hyoscine butylbromide (Buscopan), for pain
- Laxido, a laxative to control constipation caused by morphine-based medication
- Morphine sulfate (MST Continus) tablets, a potent painkiller
- Morphine sulfate oral solution, for breakthrough pain
- An atypical agent, to try to control pain
- Omeprazole, to protect stomach lining and prevent acid reflux
- Ondansetron, a strong antisickness medication
- Paracetamol, a painkiller
- Peptac, to help with acid reflux
- Prednisolone, a steroid medication

- Betnesol mouthwash dissolvable tablets, a steroid mouthwash to treat mouth ulcers
- Lidocaine 5 percent ointment, a topical anaesthetic applied to the tail end to control pain from anal fissure
- Nutritional drinks (Ensure), to maintain nutrition and energy levels

Now, that's a lot of medication to get your mind around. I went from hardly ever needing any medication to being on a long list of medications.

I was certain that the character of my pain was identical to what I had experienced when I had confirmed strictures in the past. Nevertheless, I was discharged in May 2015 on the medications listed above after investigation excluded further strictures.

My symptoms did improve somewhat after discharge, but I remained very weak and had been significantly deconditioned by this episode. Moreover, I was suffering from headaches and nausea, which were side effects of the potent medications I was on.

To make matters worse, I was advised during this very same admission that I had developed avascular necrosis of my left hip (an incidental finding on a previous outpatient MRI scan). Avascular necrosis (AVN) refers to inadequate blood supply causing death of bone tissue. The destruction of the bone ultimately results in its collapsing, requiring surgical replacement of the joint. The most likely cause in my case was use of steroid medication.

This concerned me deeply. I was now also facing the prospect of a hip replacement. On the one hand, I needed steroids to control my

Crohn's, and on the other hand, my hip was getting badly damaged. I appeared to be in a no-win situation.

I was reviewed by an orthopaedic surgeon on the ward and was advised that the consultant wished to follow up with me on a semi-urgent basis. In any case, I was obviously not fit enough for any form of surgical intervention in view of my Crohn's. I was concerned that continuing with steroids would further damage my left hip, but I appeared to have no option. The senior orthopaedic surgeon advised that it was clear the Crohn's was the acute issue that needed to take priority. If my condition remained as it was, then it was unlikely that I would have been in a position for any surgical intervention for my left hip. I would need to be stable before any surgery would be considered. It was a fine balance, but ultimately steroids were needed to control my Crohn's disease.

After discharge from the hospital in May 2015, I was reviewed by an orthopaedic specialist after completing my course of steroids. He arranged a specific MRI scan, as a matter of urgency, of both my hips to assess the extent of damage to my left hip.

To my horror, when I got the results, I discovered that I had developed extensive avascular necrosis of both hips, most likely secondary to steroid use. I was advised that I would now need to have both hips replaced at some point in the future, and that is how this will progress. My hips could collapse at any time. I was offered bone decompression surgery, but with no guarantees.

Bone decompression is a surgical procedure that is basically aimed at trying to encourage development of new blood supply to the affected bone in an attempt to prevent collapse of the joint.

Unfortunately, at the time of diagnosis, both my hips were already extensively affected, and my orthopaedic surgeon did not know if it would work or make me even worse.

If I were to go ahead with this surgical intervention to both hips, I would have to be wheelchair-bound for six weeks postoperatively. The procedure came with risks but no guarantee of success.

I had to make a decision if I wanted to go ahead with this surgical intervention for my hips, while trying to stay on top of my Crohn's disease. I was advised to take some time to come to a decision.

I decided not to go ahead with surgery. Bone decompression was not a cure, and I had concerns that my mobility would potentially be worse after surgery. At least I was relatively pain-free and mobile at present. Moreover, I had not even recovered from my last admission with Crohn's, let alone be in a position to undergo hip surgery.

This, in my mind, turned out to be the right decision, looking at matters retrospectively, as you will find out.

I was further advised by the orthopaedic specialist that I needed to be careful with any weight-bearing exercise and should refrain from even light jogging. I could not envisage being in a position to participate in any form of sporting exercise, including football, which I used to play often.

So, now I had severe Crohn's disease, which was difficult to control, possible visceral hypersensitivity, and I faced the prospect of having to undergo major surgery to replace both my hip joints at some point in the future. Surely it couldn't get worse than this? Unfortunately, it could and did get worse.

My Crohn's disease was not planning to stay quiet for long.

Unfortunately, I was readmitted in July 2015 with severe abdominal pains yet again. It was the same as before—excruciating pain, especially after eating. Again, this was very distressing for my family, watching me in so much pain. This time a CT scan confirmed an inflammatory stricture with some evidence of chronic inflammation and scarring. This made me wonder whether the recent small-bowel MRI (on the previous hospital admission) simply failed to detect the strictures I had. Although I was reluctant to take any more steroids to avoid further damage to my hips, I had no option but to restart steroids.

Despite aggressive medical treatment, my pain was only worsening. It was so severe that people who came to visit me could hear my cries of pain in the ward and left without visiting, as they could not bear to see me in so much pain. The pain kept recurring again and again until it reached a point where surgery was the only option.

I underwent major bowel surgery again to correct the strictures in August 2015, at a time when my wife was heavily pregnant with our third child. Postoperatively, I remained very unwell, in high dependency. Things just were not improving satisfactorily. My heart rate and breathing rate were high. I was in so much pain. Every day felt like a year, every hour like a day, every minute like an hour, and so on. My eyes were opening and closing. I could not communicate properly with my family. I was exhausted.

Each day after my surgery, we waited for an improvement. However, things appeared to be heading in the opposite direction instead. We all wondered why I was not recovering as expected. Things were about be explained.

Several days after this operation, while I was in high dependency, my abdomen continued to swell, and eventually brown fluid started seeping through my wound. I knew something was majorly wrong. I called the nurse, and she requested an urgent surgical review. The surgeons requested an urgent CT scan, which revealed that there was a leakage inside my abdomen. The waste from my intestine was gathering up inside in my abdomen—no wonder I felt so awful in the days after my operation. I was septic—I had a severe infection. I was struggling to breathe. My body was trying to compensate to keep me alive. My life was in grave danger.

My family were called and they visited me. I did not know if I would survive. I was so unwell that I could not think straight. My family were gathered around me. We were all distressed.

Before I knew it, I was rushed to the operating room, within a week of my last major operation, for life-saving surgery. This involved reopening my whole abdomen and washing out the contaminated contents, cutting out the damaged bowel, and forming a stoma, as it was too risky to make another joint in the bowel inside my abdomen. This life-saving operation took approximately five and a half hours. My wife and family were waiting anxiously by the phone for any news. All that my family could do was hope and pray that the surgery would be a success and that I would survive.

After the operation, I remained on ventilator support and was not awakened from anaesthetic, to allow my body to rest overnight in intensive care.

When I regained consciousness, I was in such horrific pain that I was started on three different infusions of potent medication simultaneously, administered through my veins into my bloodstream, in an attempt to control my pain. I required regular input from the specialist pain management team in hospital.

I had central lines inserted, then removed, and then reinserted due to ongoing serious ill health. I had PICC lines inserted twice.

A central line involves using a large vein in the neck to effectively administer medication directly into the main bloodstream. This requires insertion of a catheter into the vein. PICC stands for peripherally inserted central catheter, which utilises one of the large veins in the arm, allowing administration of long-term treatment such total parenteral nutrition (feeding through the veins, as in my case), chemotherapy, or prolonged antibiotic courses.

I had a large, gaping, gruesome open abdominal wound (about twenty centimetres across), which was left to heal on its own. I had two drains coming out of my abdomen draining unwanted contents from inside. I had a urinary catheter to drain and monitor urine output. I remained in the intensive care unit. I was extremely unwell.

I was fighting for my life.

Postoperatively, my bowel stopped working: I developed a paralytic ileus. This refers to paralysis of intestinal muscles resulting in obstruction of the intestine.

This caused further severe internal pain. I was vomiting foul-tasting, green-coloured bile. I could not eat and struggled to even sip fluids. My nausea was worsened by the strong pain relief medication I was on. The medication was needed for pain, but was also slowing my gut as a side effect. It was a horrible vicious cycle.

I was losing a lot of weight. I required to be fed through my veins (total parenteral nutrition) then via a nasogastric tube, which is a tube inserted through the nose into the stomach, a very unpleasant experience.

Amid such extreme circumstances, I also had to somehow come to terms with having a stoma (ileostomy) and managing it. There were times when the stoma's contents would leak into my wound adjacent to it. You can imagine the difficulties this created and the serious risk of further wound infection.

Additionally, the potent medication was making my mind feel numb. I could not get comfortable in my hospital bed. I was feeling hot and cold. My back was aching. I could not sleep.

Those were lonely, difficult times. The next few weeks in the hospital were the worst time of my life.

So many thoughts were going through my mind:

What has happened to me?
How would I ever recover from this?

How would I cope with a stoma and at the same time manage a large, open abdominal wound?

How would I possibly become well enough to start maintenance treatment for Crohn's? There were so many potential risks, especially with an unhealed wound.

What if I need more surgery to replace both my hips?

How will I be able to function?

How would I possibly be able to get back to work?

How would I support my family?

How will I be there to support my wife, who was expecting our third child?

How would my children cope with seeing me so weak and ill?

I felt like I was not in control of my body. My parents, brother, and sisters all supported me throughout, and I am so grateful to them for this. My wife travelled to and from the hospital on countless occasions to support me whilst trying to maintain some form of normality for our two young children at the same time. She was run off her feet.

I required a lot of family support. I felt upset and helpless at how my wife had to do all the running around whilst being heavily pregnant. This was a time that she needed my support, but I was not able to provide it due my ill health. I found this incredibly frustrating.

I was suffering from significant side effects of the potent medications I was on. I remained in the critical-care ward for weeks on end.

I was becoming very emotional. I pleaded with my surgeon to help me get home, at least for a few hours on a day pass to see my children. My surgeon was excellent and put a plan in place, working towards getting me home. Eventually, I was allowed home on a day pass. This made me realise how ill I was. I was taken home in a wheelchair. At this point I still had a nasogastric tube from my nose to my stomach, which was used to feed me. I struggled even to get into the car, despite help from my family. Even the slightest movement in the car caused significant pain. On arriving home, I struggled to get up the few stairs to the house. I was so exhausted that I had to lie down for most of the time at home. My body struggled to cope with even this amount of exertion. To make matters worse, the contents of my stoma leaked, causing me significant embarrassment. I had to attend to my stoma, which I found difficult and tiring, as I was not very efficient with this as yet. I realised how ill I was and how much help I actually needed.

Nevertheless, despite all these difficulties, it was all worthwhile to spend some precious time with my children.

After a long and complicated admission of almost two months, I was discharged from the hospital. I felt battered and bruised. My arms had swollen and felt like pin cushions, with the never-ending blood samples taken and the difficulties in obtaining intravenous access.

I was taken home in a wheelchair, exhausted and traumatised by the whole experience. I had to come to terms with having a stoma and a massive gaping abdominal wound adjacent to it. I struggled to breathe and could barely walk a few yards without getting short of breath. I had to take nutritional drinks to supplement my diet. I was suffering severe headaches and was dehydrated due to high stoma output. In other words, I was losing a lot of fluid through my stoma.

This was a matter of survival. I was still fighting for my life after discharge from the hospital. My family and children were upset at how weak, frail, and vulnerable I looked. There were many times when I fell asleep mid-conversation due to the drowsiness as a side effect of medication that I was taking. I was so drowsy (on the potent medication that I required for pain relief) and exhausted that I even spilt cups of water and tea on myself accidentally without warning. One minute I could be drinking water or a cup of tea and the next minute I would fall asleep, spilling the contents on myself. I was not physically capable of even the most minor tasks of daily living. I had several occasions where I felt that I was about to collapse after taking a shower. I was out of breath on minimal exercise. I was struggling to manage my stoma at first, and this really affected me. Additionally, I had to manage a large gaping open abdominal wound which required regular wound care and dressing applications with help from the district nurses, who visited me at home. I didn't even have the energy or strength to pick up my own children. I had to take regular nutritional drinks to keep my energy levels up. My whole body was severely deconditioned. I had no strength. I felt extremely unwell.

I have only really mentioned the tip of the iceberg with regard to what I went through in the hospital. I do not think that I can fully put into words the extreme difficulties that I endured. The excruciating pain, the nausea, the vomiting of bile, the horrible side effects of medications, countless needles getting jabbed into me for blood samples, repeated lines getting inserted into my larger veins, being catheterized, nasogastric tubes getting put through my nose into my stomach, repeated major surgeries, difficulty in breathing, leakage of stoma contents into my open wound, back pain from prolonged bed rest—I could go on and on, but I think you have at least gained some insight into the extent of problems that I endured. Even after discharge, I was fighting for survival and, ultimately, my life.

Unfortunately, the hospital admissions did not stop there. Within a couple of weeks of being discharged, I was admitted yet again in October 2015 with dehydration and severe headaches due to a combination of high stoma output and side effects of medication. After discharge, I had to think of the prospect of starting on potent maintenance medication to prevent the strictures from recurring. I was apprehensive, given the severe difficulties I encountered the last time I was on maintenance treatment. I had no choice but to start treatment despite all the significant risks, not least the serious risk of infection of my abdominal wound, which had not fully healed over.

In view of the complexity and severity of my case, I sought a second opinion from another gastroenterology specialist. He agreed that I required aggressive maintenance treatment, despite the risks, to control my Crohn's disease in an attempt to prevent recurrence of complications and need for further surgery. Although there had been many question marks along the way, he felt that my disease was certainly behaving in a way that was consistent with severe Crohn's disease.

Therefore, I was commenced on potent maintenance treatment, infliximab (known by the brand names Remicade and Remsima), as an outpatient. This treatment would be long term and required careful monitoring. It also came with a long list of risks. It turns out that this would by no means be straightforward for me either. I will discuss what happened to me after starting infliximab later in my story.

My wound remarkably healed much quicker than expected, and I began to manage my stoma more effectively. After six months of sick leave, I eventually somehow returned to work on a phased return. Despite reduced stamina and increased fatigue, I was determined to establish some normality in my life and start work. To many, this was an astonishing achievement in such a short time frame.

Year 2016

As a result of my surgery, fibrous bands (also referred to as internal scar tissue or adhesions) formed between tissues and organs, making them stick together. These adhesions can cause the intestine to kink, twist, or pull out of place, causing a bowel obstruction, which can then manifest as severe abdominal pain and vomiting. I developed a bowel obstruction secondary to adhesions and was admitted to the hospital yet again in January 2016, when I had just started a phased return to work.

Unfortunately, adhesions are unpredictable in how they affect any individual. I was informed that I could go weeks without problems, or years. Great, I thought, just another uncertainty in my life. Basically, I could develop a bowel obstruction secondary to adhesions at any point in the future. This would usually be managed by having a nasogastric tube inserted through the nose into the stomach, not being allowed to eat or drink, and having intravenous fluids—a very unpleasant experience. Ultimately, the aim would always be to try to ride the storm and let it settle without surgery. If surgery was required to relieve adhesions at any point, then it would result in even more new adhesions—again, a vicious cycle.

Nevertheless, despite everything that I had endured, I was determined to return to work the following week, and I did. My fellow medical professionals, family, and friends thought it was remarkable that I recovered to the extent that I became functional again, undertook shopping, managed my stoma, attended multiple hospital appointments, and started work concomitantly. On top of this, I was required to study extensively and sit for two separate module exams (as part of a six-month, distance-learning course in occupational medicine), which I passed at the first sitting despite my severe ill health. Therefore, I fulfilled the academic requirements to sit for the diploma in occupational medicine examination conducted by the Faculty of Occupational Medicine.

I was even determined to be present when my wife gave birth to our third child, irrespective of how awful I was feeling, just a couple of months after I was discharged from the hospital. Believe it or not, I made it—I was there to support my wife in the labour ward. This was the least that I could do, given how much she supported me through my critical illness despite being heavily pregnant. This was a motivating factor for me to get better.

CHAPTER 3

My Complex Story, Continued: How My Skin Became Allergic to Water Contact

I WAS EVENTUALLY deemed fit enough to commence infliximab treatment in December 2015, in an attempt to get my Crohn's disease under control. It was decided that I had to get started on maintenance treatment; otherwise I would be at high risk of redeveloping strictures with little or no warning signs. I have a very severe form of Crohn's disease, where I have a tendency to develop symptoms late, when strictures have already formed, putting me in significant danger. I had to accept the risks of this treatment.

Unfortunately, shortly after starting infliximab, I developed yet another serious problem, an uncommon condition called aquagenic pruritis. I became allergic to contact with water. Yes, that's right, I literally became allergic to water contact.

Aquagenic pruritis is a skin condition that typically causes extremely severe, intense, prickly itching without any evidence of a rash or skin lesion, caused by contact with water.

With the exception of my face, hands, and feet, even a tiny drop of water coming into contact with my body would cause the most intensely severe and almost painful itch you could possibly imagine, which would last up to two hours, or even longer at times.

At first I thought maybe the itch was a reaction to a soap, shower gel, or shampoo. However, I stopped using these products and the itch still occurred. Then I thought maybe it was the laundry powder, but I had been using the same one for years. I tried changing laundry powders, but again, no difference in the itch symptoms. The only common factor was the water itself. It might sound crazy, but it is true. I was in so much distress after a shower that I would pace up and down the house, rubbing my skin constantly. On one occasion, I quickly got dressed and ran out of the house into the freezing cold temperature. Unfortunately, nothing helped.

This was not a mild itch. It felt as if someone was pouring acid on my body, or I was being pricked with thousands of needles.

I got in touch with my own GP and tried antihistamine medications to control the itch, one after another after another. I tried almost every antihistamine I could think of but with no significant improvement in symptoms.

I contacted my IBD nurse specialist to advise her of the distressing symptoms of severe, intense itch on contact with water since commencing infliximab. She kindly contacted a consultant dermatologist for advice. Neither the dermatologist nor the IBD nurse specialist had ever seen anyone react to infliximab in this way. The dermatologist advised taking combinations of various different antihistamines, one after the other.

Nothing seemed to work. Combinations of high-dose antihistamines and moisturising agents proved ineffective. The dermatologist reviewed me urgently at her clinic. There was nothing to see on my skin. I was commenced on UVB light treatment three times per week for eight weeks. I had no option but to try this option, despite the risks involved.

So, what is UVB light treatment?

Also known as UVB phototherapy, this is basically light treatment, where the skin is exposed to ultraviolet light. It involves standing fully undressed, except for the genital region, which is covered, in an enclosed chamber equipped with special fluorescent light tubes allowing body exposure to certain types of ultraviolet light. Special safety goggles are worn to protect the eyes from damage from the light. This treatment is usually administered in a dermatology department, supervised and monitored by a specialised team of healthcare professionals. It is also used for patients severely affected by various skin conditions, including psoriasis and eczema.

However, there is a risk of the skin burning and also a risk of skin cancer.

How could I possibly live my life trying to avoid water contacting my body? Water is a basic necessity of life. Moreover, I live in a country where rainfall is so frequent and quite often predominant.

The itch was so distressing, enough to drive anybody crazy.

As you can imagine, this created enormous difficulties in my day-to-day living. I had to avoid showering as much as possible. I dreaded even a small drop of water touching my body, as it would trigger the most horrendous itch imaginable. Even when brushing my teeth, I had to make sure that my body was fully covered, since if even a drop of water touched my body anywhere other than my face, hands, or feet, it would trigger symptoms. I would have to grin and bear the distress of water touching my body for approximately one or two hours after contact. The itch was so distressing that I did not know what to do.

I live in Scotland, where rainy weather is pretty much the norm. I had to wear waterproof clothing when outdoors. Even the dampness from my clothes would trigger the most horrendous itch. I am not exaggerating by saying that water contact was like acid touching my body or like being pricked with hundreds of burning hot needles.

With a stoma that had a tendency to leak, you can only begin to imagine the difficulties involved in keeping clean when I had to avoid water contact or at least keep it to an absolute minimum.

You might find it hard to believe, but I was actually living a life where I had to try to avoid contact with water.

It was not as if I was receiving infliximab treatment every day. After my three loading doses, I received it once every eight weeks. Even if I considered stopping the infliximab, there were no guarantees that the itch would resolve. There were also no guarantees that I would tolerate alternative medication. I was stuck.

While I could not prove that my symptoms were directly due to infliximab treatment, it was highly coincidental that they started so soon after commencing this.

There was one occasion when I had to shower while in the hospital, as my stoma had leaked. I came out in severe distress. The itch was almost unbearable. I was rubbing my body up and down. I ran out into the ward to find my nurse. I was given intravenous piriton (an antihistamine) to try to alleviate my symptoms. I just had to bear the distress until it eventually settled down. This was a horrible experience.

The itch appeared to be even worse in the morning and at night, making it difficult to sleep at times.

It remains to be seen if I respond to UVB light treatment. Even receiving light treatment three times per week was exhausting. I often rushed from work, having to park and then run to the hospital to make my appointments. With all my other health issues, attending treatment on such a regular basis was physically demanding and challenging. But I had no choice.

How Have I Coped?

Despite these ongoing distressing symptoms as well as fatigue, reduced stamina, physical deconditioning, reduced exercise capacity, and the traumatic sequence of events that unfolded as a result of my complicated health issues, I was determined to continue working and getting on with my life as much as possible. Although I have had various ups and downs, I have become functional to the extent that an outsider would never be able to tell how ill I have been with Crohn's disease.

I have been told that many people would have reached breaking point and struggled to function if they had to endure what I have been through.

After reading my story about what I have had to endure, you may be thinking how I managed to become so functional and positive, return to work, and achieve such a good quality of life, which essentially appears normal to someone who does not know my history.

Well, I discovered that *the road to recovery lies within the diagnosis*, and I devised a strategy, relying on my experience as both a doctor and a patient, to optimise my quality of life. This worked for me, and I am sure it will work for any Crohn's sufferer, or indeed anyone suffering from ulcerative colitis or any other chronic illness.

My strategy to improve and optimise my quality of life is discussed in detail later in this book.

CHAPTER 4

The Impact of Having a "Disease"

SUFFERING FROM ANY chronic disease will have various impacts on a patient. I have only given my account of what has happened to me.

There is no doubt that every patient has his or her own story to tell, but I think there are certain aspects that may apply to anyone suffering with a chronic health condition, and this can affect people to varying degrees.

So, what does the word "disease" mean?

There are various definitions. However, to simplify the definition from a medical perspective, "disease" essentially refers to symptoms or signs arising from abnormalities in the structure or function of the human body. This can include various physical as well as mental health conditions.

Furthermore, I think you do not need to look any further than the word disease itself to establish how it can affect an individual.

I have relied on my experience as a patient and a doctor to summarise what I feel are the potential impacts that a chronic disease can have on a patient, either directly or indirectly. I am by no means stating that a patient will always be affected by all the points I raise, but rather that a patient might potentially be impacted by these issues. He or she might be impacted by none of these categories, one or some of the categories, or even all of the categories. The extent to which one might be affected is also variable.

Nevertheless, it is important to know how we can be impacted by disease, and here is how I have categorised it:

Disease-related symptoms/Disability
Insecurity
Social difficulties
Empathy for other sufferers
Adverse impact on psychological health
Sickness absence
Expectation that your life will never be the same

Now let us discuss each of these issues in a little more detail.

Disease-Related Symptoms/Disability

There are different ways in which disability is described. In basic terms, disability refers to a restriction in an individual's ability to undertake perceived normal activities due to one or more physical, mental, cognitive, intellectual, sensory, or developmental impairments.

Crohn's disease is no exception. It can be a severely debilitating condition that limits a person's ability to function both physically and mentally.

With reference to disease-related symptoms, any medical condition can cause either physical or psychological symptoms, or both.

Crohn's disease can cause a vast range of physical symptoms, which has been covered earlier in this book. These physical symptoms are a direct result of the underlying inflammation. It can be enough to make an affected individual housebound at times of acute flare-ups. This can have further effects on an affected individual's psychological health, resulting in symptoms of conditions such as anxiety and depression.

Imagine a Crohn's disease sufferer being unable to make it to the toilet in time when out and about. This can be a very embarrassing, humiliating, and degrading experience. This can result in anxiety on leaving the house. This can result in depressive symptoms due to not being able to do the normal things in life.

Not everybody suffers psychological symptoms, and this is just one example of how Crohn's disease can cause significant difficulties, both physically and mentally.

The point of the matter is that any disease can have a potentially significant impact on an individual's physical and psychological health.

Insecurity

Diseases such as Crohn's disease are not amenable to cure, based on current medical practice. Therefore, this is categorised as a lifelong illness that can potentially flare up at any point. This can make an affected individual go from being fully functional when in remission and symptom-free to being severely debilitated and housebound at times of relapse when symptoms are at a peak. This can naturally result in feelings of insecurity.

There are often significant financial implications as a result of job insecurity. Some organisations may not be able to sustain the level of absence that can be associated with Crohn's disease.

Even as a fully qualified and specialised doctor, I felt job insecurity given that I had such prolonged and repeated spells of absence (up to six months at a time). Crohn's disease, in my opinion, is predictably unpredictable, which can make it incredibly difficult to sustain regular employment.

There is insecurity about how the condition will progress and how this will impact both the affected individual and his or her family.

Social Difficulties

Suffering from a condition such as Crohn's disease can significantly affect an individual's social life. It becomes increasingly difficult to spend quality time with family, let alone with friends. Symptoms can render an individual housebound. Going out in public is no longer easy; it involves careful planning, identifying nearby toilet facilities, and making sure to carry spare clothing in case of an accident. Moreover, personally speaking, I found it very difficult to manage my stoma and gain confidence in managing it when out and about.

Several hospital admissions, side effects of medications, and sheer physical exhaustion can make it increasingly difficult to attain any level of social life.

I have always enjoyed my food, but with Crohn's disease I have to be careful what I eat and when at times of flare-ups. At times, due to my ill health, I have been limited in my ability to socialise with family and friends at social events.

Empathy for Other Sufferers

Even as a fully qualified doctor with experience in treating Crohn's disease patients, whilst I most certainly sympathised, I don't think I could have fully truly appreciated what it is actually like to live with such a serious condition as Crohn's disease, second by second, hour by hour, day by day, month by month, and year by year. Speaking as a patient, I believe that my treating healthcare professionals certainly *sympathise* with my health problems. However, I also believe that only another Crohn's sufferer or IBD sufferer (or someone actually living with a sufferer day in day out) can truly *empathise* and appreciate what it's like living with this condition and all the difficulties it entails. This has been a real eye opener for me.

As a Crohn's sufferer, I can now fully appreciate and put myself in someone else's shoes, and understand what it's like to live with such a debilitating condition and how it can affect not only the sufferer but also his or her family.

I have lived through and experienced, firsthand, how a condition like Crohn's disease can literally turn your whole life upside down, and before you know it, you are battling for survival.

Adverse Impact on Psychological Health

This has already been covered under "Disease-Related symptoms"; however, I am dedicating a separate heading to create awareness that any medical condition can potentially impact an individual's mental health. It is very important to be aware of this. Crohn's disease is no exception; it can potentially tear apart an individual's life causing psychological problems, and unless controlled with appropriate intervention, this can result in a vicious cycle of despair and anguish.

Not every sufferer from a physical condition necessarily develops psychological problems. Nevertheless, it can happen. Therefore, it is important to report any psychological problems to your doctor who will provide appropriate support and guidance.

I am lucky that I have always remained positive and optimistic in my approach. I believe that this attitude has been crucial in my recovery. I will talk later, in chapter 5, about the importance of positive attitude and optimism in battling through severe ill health with Crohn's disease.

Sickness Absence

It goes without saying that absence due to sickness is an inevitable result of conditions that are associated with debilitating symptoms, as is the case with Crohn's disease. I have had several prolonged spells of sickness absence as a result of my condition. Unfortunately, this was out of my control.

Sickness absence is something that is unpredictable with Crohn's disease, given its relapsing/remitting nature.

Expectation That Your Life Will Never Be the Same

Understandably, with a long-standing condition such as Crohn's disease, it is only natural to expect that your life will never be the same. In my view, this is true to an extent, but there will always be the chance to improve and optimise your quality of life and try to make the best of what you have.

How to do this will be explained in the forthcoming chapters.

CHAPTER 5

My Strategy to Improve and Optimise My Quality of Life

THE PREVIOUS CHAPTERS were an insight into my traumatic journey, the impact a disease can have, and how Crohn's disease has affected me. You must be thinking, how I picked myself up from this and got my life back on track, especially when my Crohn's was so aggressive and difficult to control with so many complications?

I needed to find a way to improve and optimise my quality of life. I soon realised that the *road to recovery lies within the Crohn's diagnosis itself.*

I applied two underlying concepts and six key principles—derived from the word "Crohn's," each letter denoting a principle—to my life and put it all together in my *hot air balloon theory,* which helped get my life back together and optimise my quality of life.

What I am going to share with you is not a cure, but rather a mechanism through which I actively helped to optimise my quality of life.

I am putting a lot of emphasis on the point that this is not a cure, but rather a strategy to help improve quality of life whilst suffering from Crohn's disease, ulcerative colitis, or indeed any chronic illness.

This is *not* a substitute for good medical care and treatment provided by your GP, family doctor, specialist, or healthcare professional. As you will see, good medical care is actually one of the foundations of my strategy, and it is imperative to maintain this crucial link and fully cooperate with your healthcare professionals, complying with their advice and treatment.

So, how does the hot air balloon theory actually work?
This involves using some of your imagination.

I imagined that a hot air balloon basket represented me as an individual, a patient suffering from Crohn's disease. If the structure of the balloon itself (that is, the envelope) is not complete and there is no hot air energy (provided by the burner), then there is no way it can make any progress getting off the ground.

I imagined that the greater the height achieved, the better the quality of life. Therefore, as it stood with me being on the ground with no structure in place (the envelope of the balloon) and no thrust of hot air energy (via the burner), my quality of life would remain low.

Therefore, I needed to make a solid structure, and I realised that this was possible through the diagnosis of Crohn's itself.

Once the structure is in place, the balloon still cannot take off unless there is a thrust of hot air allowing it to rise. Therefore, I needed to provide the thrust of energy that would allow the balloon to function.

It makes sense that both the structure and the thrust of hot air need to be in place; otherwise the hot air balloon will fail, and the basket will remain grounded.

As previously described, I imagined my quality of life being measured by the height reached by the hot air balloon (the greater the height, the greater the quality of life). The more efficiently I could get the hot air balloon working, the better quality of life I could achieve. I am not saying that I have the same quality of life as a healthy individual, but this has helped me to achieve a more optimal quality life, taking the limitations of my condition into consideration.

I got my Crohn's hot air balloon off the ground, and before I knew it, I was reaching new heights, representing better quality of life. There are six fundamental principles that I used to complete the structure of the hot air balloon and two underlying concepts to provide the thrust to get it off the ground and start making progress towards improving quality of life.

The six principles that formed the structure of the hot air balloon are all interlinked and work together to maintain the structure, and once all six principles are in place and linked together, they make a solid foundation. Each point of the hot air balloon must be intact for it to be complete in structure; otherwise it will collapse.

Now let's look at how the Crohn's diagnosis can be used to build the structure. I have referred several times to "the road to recovery lies within the diagnosis itself." I did not make this up randomly, but I gave it a lot of thought and consideration. I realised that I had become a Crohn's patient, which was out of my control. However, I thought that surely there must be a way that I could use all my medical experience as a doctor to come up with something that would positively influence my life despite suffering with Crohn's disease. And there it was, right in front of me. I was able to come up with a strategy where each letter in the word "Crohn's" denoted a principle that could be used to build a solid foundation. I would build my own hot air balloon using the very condition that I suffer from as the inspiration behind it.

So here are the six principles that theoretically form the structure (envelope) of my hot air balloon, which I will go into more detail about later. Each one of these principles has been crucial in my road to recovery.

Principle 1: **C**ommitment
Principle 2: **R**esilience
Principle 3: **O**ptimise care
Principle 4: **H**ealth/hope
Principle 5: **N**eed to accept and adapt
Principle 6: **S**upport

Here is a diagram to help visualise the structure of the hot air balloon:

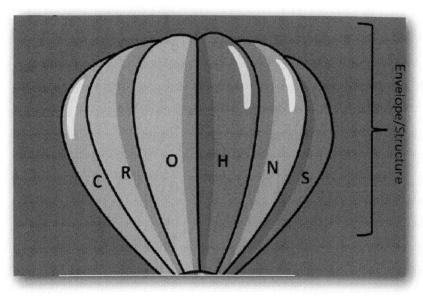

Remember that at this point, the hot air balloon remains grounded, as it is incomplete without the burner.

Now that the structure is in place, we need to look at forming the engine or burner. There are two concepts that essentially form the burner of the hot air balloon that need to be embedded in your mind. These concepts can be thought of as the thrust of hot air energy needed to get the balloon off the ground once the structure has been formed.

So, what are the two concepts that will make the burner or engine that will provide the thrust of energy to help on the road to recovery?

Concept 1: Gratitude

- Remember that there is always somebody who is worse off; therefore appreciate what you have in life, and be grateful for it.
- You may be thinking that your life cannot get worse due to your ill health, either because of Crohn's disease or any other condition. This is not true; I can assure you. Through my medical experience and patient experience, I have encountered so many different debilitating conditions. This is an eye-opener as to how much we take for granted. Take my severe reaction to water contact. Could you have even imagined that this could be possible? Most of my fellow medical professionals had never heard of this condition called aquagenic pruritis. It made me realise that I took for granted cleaning my body with water without any difficulty.
- Similarly, I have four limbs, but some people don't. I have vision in both eyes; some people don't. I can talk; some people can't. I can communicate; some people can't. I can hear; some people suffer from deafness. I can breathe; some people

have medical conditions making it difficult to breathe. The list can go on and on. The point I am making is that there are many people who are much more unfortunate than me. Therefore, be grateful for what you *do* have in life.

Concept 2: Patience

- There is no doubt that Crohn's disease has the potential to cause debilitating effects. I can vouch for that. However, the more patient you are, the easier it will get.
- Becoming impatient will only make things worse.
- Impatience will make you more frustrated, especially in chronic (long-standing) conditions such as Crohn's disease.
- Becoming more patient will help you take control of your life.

Here is a diagram of the burner (engine) of my hot air balloon and the basket that represents me as a Crohn's patient:

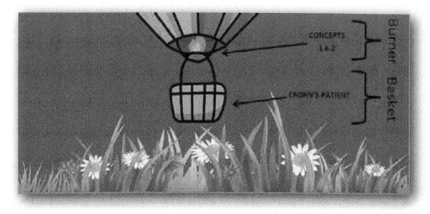

Once I built the structure of my hot air balloon using the Crohn's diagnosis and got my mind around these two concepts, my hot air balloon was ready for lift-off. As my balloon began to rise (theoretically), my quality of life started to improve, and I began to make significant progress on my road to recovery.

I am not saying that this is a cure by any stretch of the imagination. We all have different levels of quality of life that we can achieve, depending on the extent of disease and other psychosocial factors. I am also very much aware that we are here for only a limited time; however, adopting this strategy helped me progress towards my own optimal quality of life.

I incorporated this into my life, and this has helped me profoundly through my battle with Crohn's disease and its associated complications. At the end of the day, we only live once, so why not try to make the most of what we have? That's the way I look at it.

I needed to ensure that I did not fall into the vicious cycle of despair and anguish, but rather build my own hot air balloon and get it off the ground. This strategy was key for me to do whatever I could to improve my quality of life.

My Complete Hot Air Balloon Theory, Illustrated and Simplified

In this section, I will try to illustrate and simplify my concept. The purpose is to reinforce what I have just discussed and hopefully make it even easier to understand.

A hot air balloon has three main components:

1. The envelope, which comprises the actual fabric of the balloon;
2. The burner, which is effectively the engine providing hot air for the balloon, allowing it to rise; and
3. The basket, which is attached to the balloon.

Now let me try to put this into perspective.

Imagine that the basket represents you as a patient—in other words, imagine that you are standing in the basket.

Now imagine that the envelope (the fabric) of the balloon is made up of the six principles of my CROHN'S strategy: commitment, resilience, optimise care, hope/health, need to accept and adapt, and support. These six principles are required to make a robust envelope.

Even with you in the basket and a sound structure in place by applying the six principles, the balloon still requires hot air to rise.

Now think of the two underlying concepts of *gratitude* and *patience* as the burners that provide the hot air.

Once all three fundamental components of the balloon are in place, it will rise.

Now consider the height the balloon reaches directly correlates with your potential quality of life.

It is my opinion that this can represent reaching your optimal quality of life using my strategy.

To summarise, this is what I did to improve my quality of life:

- I used the six principles to build the envelope (fabric) of my balloon.
- I placed myself in the basket, theoretically speaking.
- I used the two underlying concepts in my strategy to build the burners that power the balloon with hot air.

My hot air balloon began to rise in direct correlation with my quality of life.

I hope that makes sense. The strategy can be illustrated by my hot air balloon theory as follows:

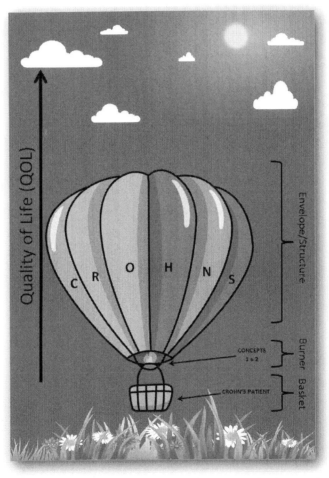

Please take time to understand this diagram. This hot air balloon theory is there to be utilised, and it has worked profoundly for me. This diagram is a summary of my strategy at a glance. Please refer to this diagram as and when required to help you understand and visualise my concept.

Let me take you through each of the six principles I used to build the envelope of my hot air balloon, which set the foundation for a better quality of life.

Principle 1: Commitment

For those suffering from Crohn's disease, you have a choice. You can either let your condition get the better of you or you can take it in your stride.

You will undoubtedly encounter difficulties and challenges through your illness. It may seem that things are spiralling out of control and your quality of life is deteriorating, and it may seem that there is nothing you can do about it.

This is wrong!

No matter how severe your condition, there is always the potential for a better quality of life.

You need to be committed to improving your own quality of life through your illness. You need to be dedicated to improving your quality of life. Yes, there will be some limiting factors that are out of your control, such as how your disease responds to medical treatment, but you need to be committed to getting on track to your own recovery.

Your quality of life will not improve to its full potential unless you are 100 percent committed to getting yourself better and improving your own quality of life.

I am not saying that there will not be highs and lows, but you need to have 100 percent commitment, for the benefit of yourself and your loved ones.

How can you become committed?

Think of the most precious things that you have in life.

Make a commitment to yourself that you will do whatever it takes to hold on to the most precious things you have by doing your part in not letting your illness dictate what you can or can't do.

For me, some of the most precious things that I have are as follows:

- My family. I want to be able to help look after my parents, who are getting older, and spend more time with them. I have a wife and three young children to support. I would like to spend as much quality time with my family as possible.
- My career. I wish to continue practising as a doctor, something that I have worked hard for all my life. Moreover, I developed an interest in occupational health medicine and wish to pursue this further.

Principle 2: Resilience
This follows naturally from Principle 1.

You need to become thick skinned, start taking things on the chin, take things in your stride, or whatever you wish to call it.

If you hit a low point, don't let it stop you from moving forward. This might mean moving forward in short bursts when your condition is more stable.

From my own perspective, I had prolonged hospital admissions and major surgeries, which meant I literally could not do anything at times. However, as soon as my condition stabilised slightly, I began to move forward.

If you give up as soon as you hit a low point, then a negative vicious cycle will ensue.

So start becoming more resilient. Always think this is not going to get the better of me.

Principle 3: Optimise Care

For a Crohn's patient, there will always be a multidisciplinary approach to care. In other words, there will be various different medical professionals involved in your care. From my own perspective, through my illness and associated complications, I have had input from the following healthcare professionals:

- General practitioner
- Gastroenterologist for investigation and ongoing medical management
- Colorectal surgeon
- IBD nurse specialist
- Stoma nurse specialist

- District nurses for wound care
- Dietician
- Anaesthetist
- Acute pain management team
- Cardiologist
- Neurologist
- Orthopaedic surgeon
- Nursing staff on medical, surgical and critical-care wards
- Physiotherapist
- Dermatologist

All these specialties were either directly or indirectly related to my Crohn's in one way or the other.

As Crohn's patients (or indeed any patients), we are the ones directly affected by our condition and suffering. Therefore, we need to take responsibility and make sure that we receive the best possible medical care and give ourselves the best possible chance for recovery. As a fully qualified medical doctor with years of experience, I cannot emphasise enough the importance of being compliant with your treatment plan as guided by your treating clinicians, doctors, and healthcare professionals.

Ways in which we can optimise our own care include the following:

- Ensure that you are happy and comfortable with the medical professionals who are treating you. It is vital that you have confidence in your doctors. If you are not confident in your doctors, then try to communicate with them to eradicate any misconceptions and build confidence. Remember, you are entitled to request a second opinion if you are still not happy.

- Become involved in your treatment and care. While it is important to allow medical professionals to do their job, it is just as important to discuss any problems, issues, or concerns you have about treatment. For example, if you have side effects to a medication, communicate this to your doctor. There may be a simple remedy to alleviate the side effects.
- Make the most of your appointments. I know, as a doctor and especially as a general practitioner, that we are under increasing pressure and demands, resulting in less time for patients. As a patient, you can optimise your time with doctors by planning your appointments. Arrive on time, have your questions written down, and express your concerns and issues succinctly. Do not be afraid to ask questions.
- Be compliant with medications.
- Keep in touch regularly with your healthcare professionals.

What did I do to optimise my care?

- I obtained a second expert opinion for my gastroenterology care in view of the complexity and severity of my disease and how difficult it was to control. I have received excellent care from both gastroenterologists involved.
- I informed my GP of the severe itching that I developed after starting infliximab and was tried on various antihistamines for this. When antihistamines failed, I did not give up and ask to withdraw from infliximab. I was aware of how crucial it was for me to try to tolerate this treatment, otherwise there could be serious consequences. Therefore, I informed my IBD nurse of the severity of my symptoms of aquagenic pruritis after starting infliximab. This resulted in an urgent referral to dermatology, and I am now receiving UVB light

treatment to control my symptoms. The dermatology team are trying their best to support me on infliximab, which I desperately need to control my Crohn's disease.

- I felt physically deconditioned after my hospital admissions and asked for a GP referral to physiotherapy to build up my muscle strength. I fully cooperated with physiotherapy and embarked on my own exercise regime to rebuild my strength and power. To look at me now, nobody can tell how ill I have been.

- Postoperatively, I tried to build on my nutrition with an appropriate diet supplemented with nutritional drinks (guided by a dietician). I knew how important it was for me to have good nutrition to improve wound healing, rebuild my strength, and increase my weight.

- I was struggling with my stoma. I was having problems with leakage, which I found embarrassing, to say the least. This was affecting my confidence. I communicated with my stoma nurse specialist, who advised me to take loperamide (to slow the bowel) and advised on products to solidify the contents in my pouch. I was still struggling with emptying my bag and hygiene issues, so I discussed this further with my stoma nurse, and I was changed to a two-piece system, which suits me far better. I still keep in regular contact with my stoma nurse. I also mentioned the high-output stoma to my colorectal surgeon, who added codeine, which also helps manage my stoma. The key point is that I communicated with healthcare professionals to try to improve my quality of life. Rather than suffer in silence, I reached out for any help that was available to me, and I persevered. I was not afraid to keep reaching out for help whenever I needed it.

Get organised, and adopt a proactive approach to your health care:

- I bought a diary to keep track of all my hospital appointments to ensure that I did not miss any. I had to become organised, otherwise the number of appointments would be out of control, especially with the complexity of my health issues.
- During hospital admissions, I would ask to speak to a senior doctor if I had any concerns.
- In view of the complexity of my condition, I kept up-to-date letters with me when I was in accident and emergency so that the doctors treating me could be as informed as possible of my situation.

As a qualified doctor, I fully appreciate the expectations and demands of the job. Sometimes demands can be overwhelming and there is simply not enough time or resources to spend more time with patients, even though we would like to do so.

Therefore, I have come up with some tips relying on both my professional medical experience and my personal experience as a patient. This puts me in a unique position to give practical and realistic advice.

It is imperative that you optimise every single outpatient appointment you have with your doctor. As patients, we can benefit from this immensely. Our time with doctors and medical professionals is limited, so we need to make sure we are in the right frame of mind to make the most of it. Here are my top ten tips to optimise your consultations. These will also give you some insight into the doctor's perspective.

Ten tips on how to optimise your consultations with doctors:

1. Do not become a "DNA" statistic; that is, "did not attend." Unless there are genuine unavoidable circumstances resulting in a DNA, it does not reflect well on us as patients if we fail to attend without a valid reason or out of lack of care and attention. There is nothing more frustrating for health professionals than appointments getting wasted as a result of DNAs. These appointments could be used by other patients who are in desperate need of care. It wastes time and resources. I think the least we can do as patients is turn up for our appointments. If for any reason you are unable to attend an appointment, get in touch with the relevant department and ask to be rescheduled. Even if you do miss an appointment and could not cancel, then out of courtesy call and explain the situation. The consultation is a two-way system in which both doctors and patients need to cooperate. Cooperation on this front will help build trust in the doctor-patient relationship.

2. Plan your appointment well in advance. I would recommend keeping a diary. I was inundated with appointments, and it was easy to lose track. If I did not keep a diary, then I would have been overwhelmed with the number of appointments I had to attend, especially when trying to get around work and family commitments.

    Make sure travel arrangements are in place and know where you are going. Enquire about parking facilities if you drive. If you are unsure, then phone and ask. This will ensure less stress on the day.

3. Arrive on time. You will not do yourself any favours by arriving late. You may not get seen, which will cause inconvenience for you. Even if you are seen after arriving late, you might cause a clinic to run behind and put unnecessary pressure on

the doctor. Think about it this way: if a doctor has twenty patients and each patient is three minutes late, this will result in the doctor finishing one hour late. Arriving on time will get your consultation off to a good start.

4. Write down your questions, as it can be difficult to remember everything you need to ask during the consultation.

5. Express your concerns clearly and concisely.

6. Take someone with you for support if you need it.

7. Stay calm, even if the clinic is running late. It is quite often not the doctor's fault. Sometimes doctors have to deal with emergencies or complex cases and require additional time. We, as patients, would also expect our doctors to spend the appropriate length of time with us to deal with any complex issues. If you get frustrated or lose your composure, it will make your consultation less productive. Try to allow for extra time when planning ahead. Remember, it only takes one complex case to delay the whole clinic. If you arrive on time, you will get seen.

8. Take a list of your current medications. This can make things a lot easier for the doctor and make the consultation more productive, which will benefit you.

9. Ensure that both your personal details (name, date of birth, address, etc.) and your GP's details are updated and correct when attending hospital appointments. Communication between primary and secondary care is crucial to maximise the quality of your health care. I am fortunate to be able to explain my health issues without difficulty because of my medical background, but this may not be the case for non-medics. Sometimes non-medics can misinterpret information, therefore it is crucial that all healthcare professionals involved in your care communicate with each other. If your GP's address is not updated, it can disrupt this vital communication

between the hospital and your community doctor. If your personal address is not updated, this can result in missed appointment letters.

10. Remember, you are the patient, and your health is the priority. In the unlikely event that you are unhappy with your care or have concerns, then you are entitled to raise these issues to resolve the situation. You are also entitled to seek a second opinion. It is important that you have confidence in your treating clinicians.

Principle 4: Hope/Health

Never lose hope. You are not alone. Remember the two underlying concepts: be grateful for what you have, and be patient. Even when I lay helpless in the critical-care wards, I always had an inner hope that I would get better, and I did.

I believe that at least 50 percent of the battle is psychological. You need to have the right frame of mind to deal with this condition.

Look after your overall health. Crohn's disease is hard enough to live with on its own; the last thing you want to do is develop other potentially preventable conditions. To do this, I would advise improving your lifestyle, after seeking specific medical advice from your own doctor, as follows:

- Stop smoking.
- Abstain from alcohol.
- Undertake regular exercise.
- Follow a controlled diet on the advice of a dietician.

- Avoid any foods that might trigger your Crohn's disease. In particular watch out for highly spiced and greasy fried foods.
- Try to enjoy doing the normal things in life; start small and build up. Despite my hip problems, I still undertake light walking and upper-body exercises in an attempt to improve my physical fitness.
- Try to take on less stress. Delegate tasks that can be delegated. Take time out to look after yourself. Participate in activities like walking or sports to keep yourself occupied, but obviously only as much as your condition allows. Simple things like avoiding long wait times in traffic by planning your journey beforehand can make a difference. We all have responsibilities in life, but I am sure you will agree that we could all take time out to do the things that we enjoy. It might be easier said than done, but try taking things in your stride and smile. In fact, believe it or not, smiling itself can help relieve stress.

How Physiotherapy Helped Me

My body was severely physically deconditioned as a result of major surgeries in quick succession coupled with prolonged hospital admissions and recovery times. I was also facing the prospect of further surgery down the line to reverse my stoma. However, I, along with my treating clinicians, was fully aware that I needed to rebuild my nutrition and strength to be in a position for further surgery. In fact, I needed to recondition my body to get some normality back in my life. Therefore, I needed expert help, and that's where physiotherapy came in. I went into a very gradual training regimen to recondition my body to get back into some form of functional ability.

My physiotherapy actually started the first day after my surgery. I required assistance even to sit up on my bed, then get to the side of the bed, then stand, then take a step, then walk with support, then eventually walk without support.

After discharge, when I was stable enough, I attended physiotherapy once a week over several months and performed various home physiotherapy exercises, and managed to achieve a level of function where I was able to attend work more regularly as my stamina and strength improved. I still continue with physiotherapy exercises.

Principle 5: Need to Accept and Adapt

It is imperative that you accept, first of all, that you suffer from Crohn's disease. There are no two ways about it; if you suffer from Crohn's disease, then you suffer from Crohn's disease.

For myself, it was a devastating diagnosis, especially as I already had five strictures in my small bowel at the time of diagnosis.

In my experience, the quicker you accept it, the quicker you can move on. Remember that life is limited. Therefore, we have to try and make the most of it.

Once you have accepted that you suffer from Crohn's disease (obviously after you have been diagnosed by a specialist), you need to adapt your life to accommodate it, rather than let it get to you and ruin your life.

Having a stoma was a major difficulty for me. It shattered my confidence at first. Initially, I thought there would not be any quality of life with it. However, I soon realised that I am stuck with it, until such time that my condition becomes stable, and the stoma can be reversed.

So I became proactive and adapted my life so that I could be as functional as possible with my stoma. I worked closely with my stoma nurse specialist and experimented with different pouches until I found the right one.

I decided that a two-piece system worked better for me. This meant I could dispose of used pouches and apply new ones. I tried different ways of changing the flange to minimise time and mess. I used a larger pouch overnight to prevent leaks and smaller pouches throughout the day generally.

I did not attend any social gatherings without having my stoma care products. If I was going to be out longer, then I would use the larger pouch to buy some time. I would always make myself aware of where the nearest toilet facilities were in case I needed to attend to my stoma.

I had to adapt the clothing that I wore to accommodate my stoma. I had a problem where I could not tuck my stoma inside my trousers, as this would simply create obstruction to the flow and cause leaks. I found it very difficult to even button my trousers due to the stoma. I only really wore tracksuit bottoms (sweatpants) for months, as I had totally lost confidence in wearing trousers. I could not tuck my shirt in, as my stoma pouch was in the way. When I recommenced work, I had a dilemma: how on earth could I dress smart and feel comfortable in my clothes at work? This forced me to adapt.

I went shopping. I managed to find smart trousers with an elastic waistband, providing some flexibility. This was ideal. Then I managed to find a smart jumper (sweater) with a collar and sleeves sewn in, making it look like a shirt underneath a jumper. The advantage of this was that the jumper would easily cover my stoma from the top without needing to tuck in the shirt.

There are many such examples that I could give about my stoma care, but the underlying point is that I adapted my life to accommodate the stoma.

I had to adapt to a variety of situations, not just to my stoma. For example, I was suffering pain in my Achilles's tendons. I did not let this put me off. I purchased shoes with air cushions to provide the extra comfort I needed. I sought advice from the physiotherapist. Sitting in a low down position or for prolonged periods would cause hip pain and pressure around my stoma region causing discomfort; therefore, I adapted by using seats with adjustable heights and took regular breaks. I asked for adaptations at work, such as extra mid-session breaks to allow time to manage my stoma. My employer was very supportive and provided any necessary adaptations thus improving my chances of sustaining work.

The point I am trying to get across is that you need to get out there and make the necessary adaptations to your life to help you move on.

Most Crohn's sufferers have good and bad days. You need to adapt your thinking. Mentally prepare yourself that you have a chronic condition that could potentially flare up at any time, but don't let it get to you and keep moving forward. Make the most of your good days. Try to find something to look forward to on your bad days—this could be something as simple as phoning a friend or family member. Always try to look at the positives, even on your bad days.

There is nothing to gain from dwelling on negatives.

You can only imagine the difficulties I faced when my body became allergic to water contact. This profoundly affected my day-to-day living. All my life I had showered every single day, and now I was in a position that I could not tolerate water touching my body. So how did I deal with it?

I accepted the fact that I needed my infliximab treatment, in the hope of preventing further potentially life-threatening episodes. There was no way around it. I knew that there was a chance I could react even more adversely to alternative treatments, given my history.

Therefore, I had no choice but to persevere with infliximab. I continued to receive whatever treatment possible from health professionals, including approximately eight weeks of UVB light treatment and strong antihistamines. Nevertheless, I still had to adapt my daily routine to adjust. I restricted my showers to once weekly and only as needed. I tried to wear waterproof clothing outdoors to avoid water contact to my affected areas (my whole body was affected except hands, face, and feet). I made sure I was fully covered for simple tasks such as brushing my teeth, to avoid drops of water splashing on my body. That's how severe it was. Even a drop of water would trigger the most horrendous, almost painful itch you could imagine. Nevertheless, I adapted my lifestyle so that I could keep moving on with my life, whilst doing everything possible to get this condition treated.

I am not saying it was not difficult, but I made ongoing efforts to adapt in order to optimise my quality of life.

I used the time that I was in the hospital for infliximab infusions (up to four hours at a time) to study for my exams for a distance-learning course so that I could keep on track to gain my diploma in occupational health medicine. I passed both exams on first sitting.

Even when I lay helpless and in extreme distress in the hospital, I still managed to arrange for a mitigating circumstances application to be submitted so that I could sit for my exam when fit to do so. I was committed to continue in my career and remained resilient throughout.

So the key point is to *accept and adapt*. You will be surprised how much you can adapt when you put your mind to it.

Principle 6: Support

Crohn's disease is a long-standing complicated condition that can have devastating effects on your life. I would like to take this opportunity to thank my family, who have supported me through such challenging and traumatic times. My family's support has been crucial to my recovery.

Don't underestimate the importance of family support. Often you will need to explain your condition to your family and friends to increase their understanding of Crohn's disease. This will hopefully make them more knowledgeable about the condition, making it easier to provide support according to your needs.

My employer has also provided much-needed support throughout my illness, improving my chances of sustaining employment.

As both a doctor and a patient, I fully appreciate the multidisciplinary approach to care, which is imperative.

Throughout my illness, whether it has been directly or indirectly related to Crohn's disease, I have required help and support from various healthcare professionals. Your general practitioner or specialist can direct you towards more help and support facilities that may be available. As previously mentioned, the following healthcare professionals were involved in my own care:

- General practitioner
- Gastroenterologist for investigation and ongoing medical management
- Colorectal surgeon
- IBD nurse specialist
- Stoma nurse specialist
- District nurses for wound care
- Dietician
- Anaesthetist
- Acute pain management team
- Cardiologist
- Neurologist
- Orthopaedic surgeon
- Nursing staff on medical, surgical and critical-care wards
- Physiotherapist
- Dermatologist

The help and support provided by your healthcare professionals is key to your recovery. I am grateful for all the help and support that I have received.

I had various complications affecting other parts of my body (not just my bowel), which meant that I required input from a more diverse range of specialties than would usually be expected for someone suffering from Crohn's disease. Nevertheless, every Crohn's disease sufferer has his or her own individual experience and individual requirements for medical input depending on the situation.

There are many useful resources online, including forums, for Crohn's disease sufferers, which can be helpful. However, it is important to be guided by your treating healthcare professionals with regard to this. Additionally, your GP or specialist team may be able to direct you to local support groups and organisations that specialise in support for Crohn's disease sufferers. Depending on your personal circumstances, it may also be worthwhile exploring if there is any financial support which you may be eligible for.

An important point to remember is:

You need to be proactive, and try to improve your own quality of life as much as possible.

If there is help and support out there, then make sure you reach out and get it!

I obviously had the advantage, due to my line of work, of pre-exisiting knowledge of what help and support was out there for me.

Even as a doctor, I still found it beneficial to communicate with other people suffering from Crohn's disease, where I could relate to their experience.

Don't hide and suffer in silence, thinking you are the only one affected. Trust me, you are not alone. In fact, you will soon realise that there are many who are much worse off than you. After I heard some stories from Crohn's sufferers, it made me appreciate what I had.

So that completes the details of the six principles that theoretically form the structure (envelope) of my hot air balloon, which should be combined with the burner (two underlying concepts of *gratitude* and *patience*) to allow it to rise in order to reach your optimal quality of life.

CHAPTER 6

Misconceptions

I AM SURE that if you are a Crohn's sufferer, you might have encountered people who are not medical professionals trying to give you inappropriate advice. Whilst their intentions may be good, they often have misconceptions about this condition. I found this to be the case myself.

One common misconception I have encountered is "your condition is there purely because of what you eat." I do not believe this is accurate. We know that the underlying mechanism of Crohn's disease is autoimmune, which means the body attacks its own cells, resulting in inflammation and other symptoms. Yes, it is true that certain foods can trigger a flare-up, and diet is thought to be a possible *theoretical* contributing factor. However, there is no conclusive evidence that diet alone actually causes Crohn's disease. Many people who had the same diet as mine have not gone on to develop Crohn's disease.

A few key points to consider are given below:

- If Crohn's disease is purely related to diet, then why are there so many people with similar diets who do not go on to develop the condition?
- There is no doubt that some Crohn's sufferers can identify certain foods or ingredients that may trigger a flare-up, but

    this does not necessarily mean that the underlying disease is directly due to diet alone. I, personally, did not identify any food triggers. However, I fully appreciate that many sufferers have identified food triggers.

- Remember, diet is thought to be a possible *theoretical* contributing factor. However, there is no conclusive evidence that diet alone actually causes Crohn's disease. The underlying mechanism is autoimmune.

I also try explaining it to people like this: imagine you have a wound somewhere on your body that was accidentally caused by a sharp object. If you were to rub salt on the wound, it would make your pain and suffering worse. Now, if someone were to say that the cause of the wound was the salt, they would be wrong. Common sense says that the sharp object is the cause of the wound, but the salt makes it worse. If there was no wound, then there would be no pain if you applied salt to the area.

It's the same concept with Crohn's disease. There is an autoimmune process that causes the underlying inflammation and damage to the gut (this is the cause of the "wound," theoretically speaking). Now think of the food you eat as the "salt"—if you eat certain foods, that could cause more suffering as the gut is already inflamed. If the gut was not inflamed, then that same food would not cause problems. That is, if there was no wound, the salt would not cause any problems.

I am not, by any means, saying that dietary control is not important. Certain foods or ingredients can certainly trigger flare-ups in Crohn's sufferers. Therefore, it is imperative to avoid food triggers and to eat according to what your condition allows, under the supervision of your treating clinicians, dieticians, or specialists. I am just trying to clarify a misconception that I have encountered, namely, that I am suffering from Crohn's disease solely as a result of my diet. It is important to understand that there is an underlying autoimmune process that causes the inflammation. This overactive autoimmune process needs to be controlled. In some cases, dietary control can help, but in many cases, appropriate medical intervention is required.

Another misconception I have come across was when I was admitted with a bowel obstruction secondary to adhesions. Adhesions are scar tissue that forms after surgery and causes internal organs to stick together; it can cause bowel obstruction, but this can be very unpredictable. Now, I had been eating and drinking normally for months after recovering from my surgery, until one evening I developed excruciating abdominal pain and was admitted to the hospital again. I found it frustrating that some people blamed what I had eaten just before the pain developed. I had been avoiding the definite nos like seeds, nuts, sweet corn and popcorn, and had eaten the exact same food many times before that evening without pain. So I thought of explaining it as follows:

Think of your intestine as a flexible pipe and food as the water flowing through it. If something presses on the pipe causing it to kink or bend, then the flow of water will be obstructed, causing back pressure and problems. Would you blame the water for this? No. You would blame the object that was causing the kink or bend, or the pipe itself (if something wrong with the pipe). If the pipe were to unbend, then the water could flow freely again.

The same concept can be applied to adhesions that cause obstruction. The problem, in this situation, is with adhesions that cause the bowel to become narrowed. The food you eat then gets stuck. If this resolves and the narrowing resolves, then that food can be eaten again, as was my case. The point of the matter is, don't blame the obstruction on the last meal when it is due to adhesions. It's not always that straightforward.

There are, of course, other causes of bowel obstruction that are internally more directly related to the food you eat. For example, nuts, seeds, sweet corn, and popcorn can cause obstruction as they are not well digested.

Some key points to remember are listed here:

- The underlying cause of bowel obstruction can be more than just the food someone eats. For example, it can be due to adhesions (scar tissue) inside the abdomen.
- My nutrition was key to my recovery. If I did not eat the food that I was allowed to eat, then I would not have been able to absorb the nutrients from it to allow the massive open abdominal wound to heal and my weight to increase after it dropped dramatically postoperatively.
- I am not recommending any specific diet here. Crohn's disease is a very individual condition, and you should always seek advice from your own treating clinician, dietician, or specialist.
- I am just trying to explain a misconception that some people had about my bowel obstruction, which was due to adhesions, as confirmed on CT scan. Sometimes there is a wider picture to look at, rather than always blaming the food that you ate.

Another misconception that I have encountered is that inflammatory bowel disease (IBD) is the same as irritable bowel syndrome (IBS). This is wrong. Although IBD and IBS both affect the bowel, they are two very different conditions that require different types of treatment.

CHAPTER 7

Transitioning from Being a Doctor to Becoming a Patient

So what's it like being on the other side? What's it like going from being a doctor to a patient?

Believe it or not, I have been asked on more than one occasion, "But you are a doctor. How can you suffer from Crohn's disease?" At the end of the day, we are still human beings and susceptible to illness just like any other person. Yes, it is important to have awareness and reduce the risk factors for disease, but it can still happen to anyone.

As a doctor, I have always been used to investigating and treating patients with various conditions, including Crohn's disease. I have always sympathised with my patients; however, this experience has given me insight into what it actually means to suffer from such a debilitating condition. I am now able to empathise with other sufferers.

People often say to me that it must be worse being a doctor and that you should forget being a doctor when you are a patient. Yes, it can be frustrating as a doctor when things are not done to the standard you would expect, and it is difficult to ignore any inadequacies you may encounter as a patient. Although I have received some excellent care, there were many times when I had to point out inadequacies that I had picked up on. However, I don't believe that doctors, or indeed other medical professionals, need to pretend not to be medics if they become patients. In fact, it's not that easy to switch off from being a doctor when you become a patient. It's like asking a hair stylist not to notice people's hair styles, a make-up artist not to notice make-up, a chef not to notice cuisine. Obviously, it's only natural for them to do so, because that's what they do in their occupations every day. Similarly, as a medical professional, I have acquired inherent clinical skills, so there is no doubt that I will be knowledgeable when it comes to my own medical care. I actually have noticed many benefits of being a patient with a medical background. I am content about my condition and my treatment and can keep things in perspective. I am in a good position to understand my health care. I can communicate my health issues effectively to my family.

I have worked hard all my life to get to where I am. I worked hard at school to get the grades on exams to get me into medical school. I studied long and hard at medical school for five years to gain my medical degree at the age of twenty-two. I then worked long shifts during my hospital posts, including many long night shifts. I then completed eighteen months of GP registrar training to finally complete my specialty training in general practice. I then worked for years helping my patients in a general practice setting as well as an emergency out-of-hours setting.

Why should I pretend not to be a medic just because I am now the other side, dependent on the very care that I have provided for so long?

I have always expressed professional courtesy to any fellow medical professional that I might have treated as one of my patients. Similarly, most of my own treating clinicians and healthcare professionals have extended professional courtesy to me. I have always allowed medical professionals who are treating me to do their job without interfering, but I believe that I have used my medical background to positively influence my care. I have worked in collaboration with my treating medical professionals to become actively involved in my care. I think there is nothing wrong with that.

There have been times when I have guided medics about my care due to its complexity. I have been able to succinctly give a history every time I have been admitted. I was able to wean off strong pain-killers in a safe manner, just as I would have advised any of my own patients if they were in my situation. I firmly believe that I am in a better position to gauge my health status. Many times, I picked up on early warning signs and went to the hospital. At the same time, I have a clear understanding of why I am on each and every medication.

I was offered bone decompression surgery for my hips, and I was in a better position to make the decision not to go ahead with this. I understood the disease processes and had to prioritise my health, by choosing to get my Crohn's disease fully stabilised first. I made an informed decision to wait and hope with regard to my hips. My body was not ready to undergo any other surgical procedure. I used my medical knowledge to make informed and sensible decisions.

In summary, I use my knowledge and experience to my advantage. My case has been so complex, but I have been able to make sense of it all. Many of my treating clinicians have appreciated my input, and we have worked together to optimise my care.

Additionally, I have been approached many times by senior doctors in the hospital, asking if I would allow them to teach medical students using me as a subject. I have fully cooperated with my treating clinicians by giving permission for medical students to review my case and practise their clinical skills. This brought back memories of when I was a senior doctor in the hospital teaching medical students myself. I would never have imagined at that point that one day I would be lying in the bed as a patient surrounded by medical students learning from my own case. I suppose it just goes to show that you never know what's round the corner in life.

CHAPTER 8

Crohn's Disease from an
Occupational Health Perspective

MOST OF MY daytime work through my most severe ill health has been in a training occupational health role dealing with management referrals.

I find this role fascinating and feel that my specialist GP skills are transferable. In occupational health, we focus on how health can affect an individual's work and how work can impact upon health. In this post, I have a dual role for both the employer and the employee. As a GP, I have seen firsthand how being absent from work long term can adversely affect an individual's health and how getting back to work can positively influence health.

Absence from work due to long-term sickness can be detrimental to an individual's well-being both psychologically and physically, as well as unviable to the employer.

I wanted to make a positive difference in the well-being of patients, and occupational health provided me with this opportunity. In occupational health, we come across a wide and diverse range of medical issues, similar to general practice, except we are not in a treating role but more an advisory role both to employer and employee. While there are many branches of occupational health, my role mainly focuses on managing sickness absence and promoting health at work. I feel that I can positively influence the health of employees. I have to ensure that my advice will not put an employee's health at risk whilst also ensuring a safe return to work after a period of absence. We provide advice on strategies on ensuring good health at work. This is beneficial to both the employer and employee.

So you are probably wondering what made me look at a career in occupational health medicine in addition to general practice. Well, some of the reasons for this have already been outlined, but there are some other factors that made me intrigued.

As a medical student years ago, I worked part-time in various High Street retail shops to earn a little cash to keep me going. I also worked in call centre jobs besides working in the catering industry. This led to a significant interest in the business side of things. I was fascinated by how these large organisations ran so efficiently and managed their employees. Moreover, I really found it interesting to gain insight into various different occupations or jobs that were out there and how health impacted upon work, and vice versa. Occupational health gave me the opportunity to use my medical skills in a more corporate setting with large organisations, helping to manage staff sickness absence and offering opinions on fitness for work. As mentioned earlier, the advice I provide can benefit both employees and employers, thereby promoting health at work, which in turn leads to greater productivity for the company.

Through my severe ill health with Crohn's disease, I became subject to an occupational health assessment myself. In view of the complexity and severity of my condition, which has resulted in prolonged periods of sickness absence, I underwent an occupational health assessment by an independent doctor from a different company. This put me in a unique position, where the roles were reversed and I was subject to the same assessment that I would usually provide.

My personal experience as an employee returning from prolonged sickness absence gave me invaluable insight into the employee's journey through ill health, how it affects work, and the implications to the employer.

I take several learning points from my own personal experience:

- An impartial occupational health assessment is beneficial to both the employee and the employer, even though my employer is actually one of the leading occupational health providers specialising in this field.
- The occupational health advice that we received ensured that I could attempt a supported return to work without aggravating my health and without hindering my recovery phase, by giving appropriate recommendations on adaptations, adjustments, and restrictions.
- This helped set the foundation for a return-to-work plan that my employer and I were both happy with.
- This improved my general well-being and allowed me to return to work on a phased return, with appropriate adjustments (such as allocating specific breaks to attend to my stoma and being allowed to attend hospital appointments if they clashed with working hours). Therefore, I could provide

effective work during the times I was working, and would hope that I contributed to productivity for my employer.

I feel that undergoing an occupational health assessment and having to work with my own employer to establish me back at work, despite prolonged spells of absence due to ongoing health problems, has provided me with unique and invaluable insight into the very field that I work and train in.

I feel that I can empathise with both employees and employers when it comes to managing sickness absence. I know what it's like to be an employee who is keen and enthusiastic to work, but has been limited by severe ill health—in my case Crohn's disease. I also appreciate the difficulties and challenges that an employer faces when having to accommodate an employee with severe health problems.

Luckily for me, as you would probably expect, being a leading occupational healthcare provider in the private sector, my employer has supported and accommodated me remarkably well, for which I am very grateful.

I have personally experienced how much can be achieved if both the employee and employer are willing to have some degree of flexibility in working arrangements.

My personal experience will help in my day-to-day work in the field of occupational health medicine. I would like to think that my experience and journey through this has vastly increased my understanding of occupational health. I feel that I can utilise my experience to my advantage to become a better occupational health doctor in the future.

Occupational Health Principles Pertaining to Crohn's Disease at the Workplace

EMPLOYEE'S PERSPECTIVE

As an employee suffering from Crohn's disease, the impact on employment can vary widely irrespective of your profession. Crohn's disease is a very individual condition with a wide spectrum of clinical manifestations. Some sufferers may be affected minimally with minimal disruption to their working life, while others may be affected profoundly, to the extent that they require frequent and prolonged periods of sickness absence. It is a long-standing condition that follows a relapsing and remitting course, so there is a likelihood of having periods of better health when employment can be sustained and periods of poorer health when work cannot be sustained.

EMPLOYER'S PERSPECTIVE

As an employer, it is important to understand the nature of Crohn's disease and how it can impact an affected employee. It may be necessary to implement appropriate interventions, adjustments, or adaptations, such as flexible work hours and easy access to toilet facilities, to help improve an employee's chances of sustaining work. It is also important for employers to understand that Crohn's disease is an unpredictable chronic condition that can flare up at any time even with maintenance treatment. Therefore, it is important to understand that there will always be a risk of repeated sickness absence, depending on the nature and severity of the disease. For an affected employee, there may be periods of time, again variable in length, when symptoms are controlled and he or she is able to provide reliable and effective service, and there may be other times when symptoms are less controlled, resulting in reduced ability to perform at and sustain work.

Nevertheless, although there is a wide variation, quite often, both employers and employees can be cautiously optimistic that medical intervention will induce and maintain remission allowing for greater productivity in the workplace.

It is also important for both employers and employees to be mindful of any stress issues at work and seek resolution, to avoid any adverse impact on health, especially when an individual suffers from a condition like Crohn's disease, which can flare up with stress, according to some patients' experience. I am not saying that there will always be work-related stress issues. I was lucky in that my employer was very supportive, and we had a good mutual understanding so I had no work-related stress issues. However, other individuals might encounter some work-related stress issues and it is important to seek resolution for the benefit of both the employee and employer.

CHAPTER 9

How Crohn's Disease Has Changed Me as an Individual and a Practising Doctor

How Crohn's disease has changed me as an individual
I APPRECIATE EVERYTHING that I have in life, even the things that are taken for granted. I appreciate that I have eyes to see, lungs to breathe, a brain to function, arms and legs to use, kidneys that function, and the list goes on and on.

There were times when I struggled with breathing, and sometimes in life you don't appreciate what you have until things stop functioning the way they are meant to.

I value each and every minute that I have with my family and try to live life to the full, each day as it comes. I know there might be days when I will be limited due to ill health, but I try to make the most of the good days and the bad days.

Even writing this book was a challenge due to my ongoing health issues; however, I used any spare time that I had when I was feeling relatively better to slowly write my book. There were several occasions when I had to stop writing due to feeling unwell. Nevertheless, I remained resilient and motivated to write this book, which I hope other

Crohn's disease sufferers (or indeed any individuals suffering from chronic illness) will find useful.

How Crohn's disease has changed me as a doctor working in general practice

I have always maintained that working as a doctor is a privilege rather than a right. I am currently experiencing, firsthand, what it is like to be a patient suffering from a serious illness. This has made me even more determined and motivated to continue working as a doctor, trying to help positively influence the health and lives of my patients.

I am lucky to be in a position where I can help patients suffering from various medical conditions.

How Crohn's disease has changed me as a doctor working in occupational health

Again, the personal experience of being a patient suffering from a serious medical condition has given me insight into how health can affect the ability to work—and vice versa.

I feel that I have more in-depth knowledge of the challenges in sustaining work while suffering from a serious medical condition.

I feel that my personal experience as a patient has placed me in a better position to understand the implications that ill health can have on employment and how best to advise both employees and employers accordingly in my day-to-day practice.

CHAPTER 10

How My Religion Has Always Helped Me through My Ill Health

THE HOT AIR balloon strategy described in previous chapters is applicable irrespective of your background, occupation, race, or religion.

Falling ill has made me value and appreciate each and every second that I have in life, including precious time to spend with my family and loved ones.

Speaking from my own experience, my religion, Islam, has provided me with an inner peace that has helped me profoundly throughout my illness. Even during my most severe ill health, in my deepest and darkest times when I lay helpless in extreme pain in the hospital unable to talk or communicate effectively, I still found peace, tranquillity, and strength simply by focusing on my religion. As a Muslim, I believe that there is none worthy of worship except Allah (God) and that the Prophet Muhammad (Peace Be Upon Him) is the final Messenger of Allah.

Islam has taught me how having patience and expressing gratitude to Allah is beneficial both in this life and in the hereafter. Islam has taught me never to lose hope.

At the end of the day, despite my ill health, I still consider myself lucky to be alive, and I am still better off than millions of others around the world who, unfortunately, face serious adversities in life such as poverty, strife, displacement and so on.

Conclusion

ANYONE CAN DEVELOP Crohn's disease—it happened to me.

You have a choice. Either you make the most of your life or you let your disease get the better of you.

I hope my story will inspire you to take some of the same steps I did to improve your quality of life. Despite the different challenges you may encounter due to Crohn's disease or any illness, I believe that there is always room for improvement in your quality of life. However, in order to achieve this, you need to change your frame of mind.

I have many challenges ahead and there are still so many uncertainties:

Will my Crohn's disease get under control?
Will I tolerate medication?
Will I respond to treatment that will allow my body to contact water again without such severe and distressing symptoms?
Will I be able to sustain work?
Will my stoma get reversed?
Will I need to undergo surgery to my hips?
Will I achieve a diploma in occupational health medicine?

The list goes on!

Nevertheless, I remain optimistic and will continue to fight for survival through my illness every day. Who knows—I might even write another book about my ongoing journey, so look out for what happens next.

I will finish with the take-home message for this book.

The road to recovery lies within the diagnosis:

Commitment
Resilience
Optimise care
Hope/health
Need to accept and adapt
Support

Remember, have *patience* and *gratitude* for what you *do* have in life. Try not to dwell on negatives. Trust me, thinking in this way made a difference for me, and it will make a positive difference for you.

Why don't you try applying my hot air balloon strategy?

Good luck with your journey!

36673169R00072

Printed in Great Britain
by Amazon